"As a dialectical behavior therapy (DBT) therapist, I'm very excited to recommend *The Stronger Than BPD Journal* to my clients. This is a wonderful companion to Debbie's first book, and will help take readers to a place in their lives where they'll build even more resiliency and support in their recovery."

—**Amanda L. Smith, LCSW**, author of
The Dialectical Behavior Therapy Wellness Planner

"Two wise women help empower others to do a thorough inventory of all the patterns that will help you achieve equanimity."

—**Tamra Sattler, PhD, MFT**, therapist, researcher,
and entrepreneur

The
Stronger
than
BPD

Journal

**DBT ACTIVITIES TO HELP WOMEN
MANAGE EMOTIONS *and* HEAL FROM
BORDERLINE PERSONALITY DISORDER**

**DEBBIE CORSO
KATHRYN C. HOLT, LCSW**

New Harbinger Publications, Inc.

Publisher's Note

This publication is designed to provide accurate and authoritative information in regard to the subject matter covered. It is sold with the understanding that the publisher is not engaged in rendering psychological, financial, legal, or other professional services. If expert assistance or counseling is needed, the services of a competent professional should be sought.

This book is independently authored and published and is not endorsed or sponsored by or affiliated with any third party. By way of example, this book is not endorsed by or affiliated in any way with Dr. Marsha M. Linehan, who is recognized as a pioneer in the field of Dialectical Behavior Therapy.

Distributed in Canada by Raincoast Books

Copyright © 2018 by Debbie Corso and Kathryn C. Holt
    New Harbinger Publications, Inc.
    5674 Shattuck Avenue
    Oakland, CA 94609
    www.newharbinger.com

Cover design by Amy Shoup

Acquired by Jess O'Brien

Edited by Marisa Solis

All Rights Reserved

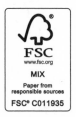
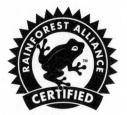

Library of Congress Cataloging-in-Publication Data on file

Printed in the United States of America

21 20 19

10 9 8 7 6 5 4 3

Contents

Part 4: Connecting, Loving, and Boundaries

Part 5: Setting Intentions and Ideas for Future Exploration

Foreword

Dialectal behavior therapy (DBT) has long stressed the presence of *Wise Mind*, an inner blend of reason and emotion that gives us direct access to our innate, intuitive wisdom. When I initially learned about wise mind, my biggest question was "But how do I *really* access it?" Sure, it's a great concept, and in rare moments, I'd become aware of that "small silent voice within." But I didn't want that voice to be small or mainly silent! I wanted and needed it to be strong, clear, and directly accessible. Wise mind needed to be a part of me, as real as my feelings and thoughts. So how does a person go from practicing the DBT skills and being "dialectical" to relying on this Yoda-like force of clarity, insight, and intuition?

Well, look no further. This groundbreaking book shows us the way. Debbie Corso and Kathryn Holt, veteran teachers and practitioners of dialectical behavior therapy, envision wise mind as a living part of us in the form of a "Wise Woman." Our Wise Woman is intuitive, ever-present, and an intrinsic part of ourselves; like wise mind, she is the union of reason and emotion. But in this book we discover that she also is so much more. Wise Woman is a presence within us; we can speak to her, call on her, and receive direct guidance from her—all of which *The Stronger Than BPD Journal* teaches us to do. The powerful and unique practices in this book guide us toward developing a relationship with that part of ourselves that serves our greatest good. And lucky for us, the techniques do not involve sitting in silence under tree all day! Instead we get to have fun, be creative, and nurture ourselves—and who wouldn't want more of that in life?

The Stronger Than BPD Journal is a brilliant road map not only because it helps us discover and connect with our Wise Woman. It recognizes that our capacity for healing and wholeness resides within ourselves. A central fact for many of us with trauma, BPD traits, and emotional sensitivity is that we are disconnected from ourselves. We have therefore also lost our connection to the Wise Woman inside us. With this book, Debbie and Kathryn help us further our journey toward reclaiming ourselves. With their help, we discover that self-trust, confidence, and self-love are all inside jobs—that is, when we know how to look and what to listen for. We understand that our deepest wisdom and enduring strength cannot be taken or given, but is our natural state, a guide that never left us and never will.

—Kiera Van Gelder, MFA
Author of *The Buddha and the Borderline*

Introduction

Do you ever feel like life is just too much to manage because you experience your emotions so deeply and intensely? Do you ever wish that you had a way to tune in to your own intuition without becoming overwhelmed? Maybe you feel as though simply navigating the world—from handling everyday tasks to managing more challenging situations—is too much to bear. You might hunger to know your place in the world as an emotionally sensitive person. No matter the cause, when your emotions come they are so intense that they affect your ability to think clearly and make wise decisions—and you end up experiencing lots of suffering.

Your suffering might appear as struggling to achieve what you deeply desire in life, such as feeling balanced and stable, handling emotional triggers without a crisis, keeping a job, or forming and maintaining meaningful relationships. These desires can feel painfully out of reach when you don't know how to manage your emotions. You may even have grown hopeless about being able to get out of this rut and build the life you really want.

But something is shifting. You're feeling motivated and want to examine the self-defeating thoughts and behaviors that have been holding you back. You're becoming curious about the strong impact of your thoughts on your mood. You're ready to change course—from living in a state of emotional reaction to skillfully responding to life's inevitable upsets. While it is not a replacement for therapy, the *Stronger Than BPD Journal* provides practices that will help you see and experience your emotional sensitivity as a strength. This journal can be a great beginning for self-exploration and healing. You are certainly not alone, and there is hope. This book is written for *you*.

Emotional Sensitivity

Maybe you have borderline personality disorder (BPD), BPD traits, or are emotionally sensitive and experience your emotions much more intensely than other people.

Borderline personality disorder is a diagnosis that is characterized by intense emotions, chaotic relationships, and difficulty tolerating distress, and these challenges persist throughout a person's life (American Psychiatric Association 2013). According to the biosocial theory of BPD, this emotional sensitivity is a result of biological disposition, living in invalidating environments, and the interaction of these factors (Linehan 1993).

Some people identify with certain traits of this diagnosis without fully meeting the criteria for BPD. This is referred to as having *BPD traits*. Throughout this journal, we use the term *emotionally sensitive* interchangeably with BPD and BPD traits.

Whether you identify as having borderline personality disorder, BPD traits, or emotional sensitivity, you may be familiar with experiencing intense, frequent, and prolonged emotions. And, as a result, you may notice challenges in the following areas of your life:

- **Relationships often feel intense, unstable, and fleeting.** There is often a strong fear of abandonment and rejection that fuels this.

- **Emotions often seem overwhelming and as if they'll last forever.** This is because people with BPD traits experience emotions for a greater period of time, causing their nervous systems to stay activated longer than a person without BPD traits. This makes it harder to return to a sense of emotional equilibrium (Aguirre and Galen 2013).

- **Behavioral responses are frequently self-harming or self-sabotaging.** Because emotions can feel so intense and, at times, unbearable, people with BPD sometimes gravitate toward impulsive behaviors that provide temporary relief despite long-term consequences.

- **Helpful coping skills are lacking.** According to dialectical behavior therapy, people with BPD or BPD traits may not have learned how to modulate their behavior in response to strong emotions. Effective skills they typically lack include self-soothing, problem solving, and focusing attention (Linehan 1993).

What Is DBT?

Dialectical behavior therapy (DBT) is a therapeutic technique developed by Marsha Linehan. It is designed to help people who experience intense, frequent emotional challenges and self-harming behaviors to live with increased freedom and self-regulation. Originally, DBT was intended specifically for women with BPD who struggle with suicidal behaviors and who were considered largely "incurable" (Linehan 1993). Since its inception in the 1990s, DBT has been modified and expanded to help all kinds of people who experience impulsive behaviors and intense emotions.

DBT is a combination of *cognitive behavioral therapy* (CBT) and Zen Buddhism. CBT forms the basis of identifying how thoughts influence emotions and behaviors, and Zen Buddhism forms the basis of learning how to be present with what is and to radically accept what shows up in any given moment. This combination of behavioral and mindfulness approaches offers a concrete way of working with thoughts and feelings while also providing practices that center the body and mind to help us connect with our own inner wisdom.

DBT Background

A basic premise of DBT is the idea that living in an "invalidating environment" increases *emotion dysregulation*, or difficulty modulating emotion intensity, by invalidating (or negating and dismissing) our emotional experience. This theoretically leads to difficulty knowing what we are feeling and how to cope with the feeling effectively. Many people who struggle with emotional sensitivity grew up or live in invalidating environments, and learning how to self-validate one's emotions—knowing what is being felt, naming it, and coping without making the situation worse—is often a primary goal of treatment.

An important viewpoint of DBT is that people who are emotionally sensitive and experience impulsivity are not inherently flawed. Rather, through a combination of biology and environmental factors, they have a "skills deficit," which simply means that certain skills were not learned during childhood and beyond. The primary missing skills Dr. Linehan and her team noticed in their clients were knowing how to tolerate distress without creating more of a crisis, being able to regulate emotions by calming down or changing emotions as needed, expressing needs and feelings in relationships, and being in the present moment (Linehan 1993).

To address these needed skills, DBT is organized into four modules that are taught in DBT groups and classes:

- Mindfulness

- Emotion regulation

- Distress tolerance

- Interpersonal effectiveness

In each module, clients and students learn concrete tools and techniques for working with their own emotions, states of mind, and relationship dynamics.

In addition to skills groups, DBT also incorporates individual psychotherapy. In individual DBT, therapist and client explore the function of problematic behaviors, practice making and sustaining a therapeutic relationship, and problem solve skills use, among many other goals the client has for individual therapy.

Much of DBT is focused on helping clients learn how emotions, thoughts, and behaviors influence one another, and how to work with each of these to build a life worth living. This is accomplished through learning new skills, practicing them in real life, and receiving validation and feedback from group members and their therapist (Linehan 1993).

There Is Hope and Help in These Pages

In this book, you'll be supported in:

- transforming your inner emotional chaos into insight, wisdom, and a feeling of connectedness to yourself, others, and the natural world;

- beginning to accept and better manage your BPD traits and emotional sensitivity as a superpower;

- creating a more-balanced life that is nourishing instead of depleting; and

- responding instead of reacting to your emotions, reducing the unnecessary suffering that can come with impulsive decisions.

When you feel ill equipped or insecure about your ability to regulate your emotions, you end up repeatedly looking outside yourself for direction and reassurance. Eventually, this becomes disempowering and leads to a lack of self-trust. This can take a toll on your self-respect and relationships, so we're going to take a radically different approach on our journey together in this journal.

We're going to look at any tendencies you may have to shift between the extremes of emotions and thoughts. We'll explore the importance of acknowledging and honoring each, along with the benefits of finding the middle gray area where you can skillfully combine and balance the two. We'll also look at how having BPD traits or emotional sensitivity makes you more susceptible to emotion dysregulation when it comes to feeling, expressing, and shifting out of intense and overwhelming emotions. You'll build your resiliency so you can handle these things with more confidence.

This journal is a road map to the destination you are ultimately seeking: the discovery and befriending of the part of you that knows how to transform your emotional sensitivity into a superpower of strength, intuition, and resiliency.

Your Inner Wisdom

The exercises in this journal are based on the primary skills modules of DBT. These skills are designed to help us live more mindfully, cope with emotional distress, avoid emotional crises, and have healthier relationships. In DBT, we practice moving among three common states of mind: emotional, rational, and inner wisdom.

The *emotional mind* is the part of you that is guided by your emotions and feelings. It experiences the full range of emotional territory, from anger to joy to love to sadness. People who are emotionally sensitive or who have BPD traits can often feel ruled by this part of themselves.

On the other end of the spectrum, you have your *rational mind*, which is the part of you that is systematic, logical, and linear. Your rational mind is like your inner computer that helps you use reasoning and planning to get from point A to point B and to solve problems.

Sometimes people get stuck vacillating between the emotional and rational states of mind—you feel overly emotional and then try to compensate by becoming "logical" and "making sense." However, this swing doesn't tend to help for very long because you ricochet right back to being overly emotional. To feel emotions and use logic *at the same time*, you need to access a deeper, more intuitive part within you. This is your *inner wisdom*; in this book, we refer to it as your "Wise Woman." She is the strong, resilient part of you who often gets lost or forgotten in an overly stimulating world, yet she is your inner compass for wisdom and discernment.

Your Wise Woman might show up as a sensation in your heart or belly as a "gut feeling," or as an intuitive, instinctual knowing. She is capable of holding both emotions and logic simultaneously without getting swallowed by intense emotions or shutting down feelings for the sake of your rational mind.

This journal is meant to help you explore the voice, resources, and insights of your Wise Woman. The exercises will help you access her wisdom. You'll begin trusting her—and calling on her again and again—through creative, fun, and perhaps challenging writing exercises. These activities serve as portals to the part of you who can guide you in making choices that are for your highest good and not based in fear or habitual reactions.

How to Use This Journal

This journal is organized into five parts:

- How to Listen to Your True Inner Voice

- Handling Life Stress, Upsets, and Triggers

- Strengthening Your Emotional Resiliency from the Inside Out

- Connecting, Loving, and Boundaries

- Setting Intentions and Ideas for Future Exploration

In each part, you'll be challenged to dig deep and allow your feelings and inner wisdom to flow through journaling. Writing is a powerful way to access emotions, thoughts, and the voice of your Wise Woman. Beyond helping you slow down and better understand your inner experiences, the act of putting feelings and thoughts into words on paper through writing or typing can help improve depressive symptoms and increase emotional regulation (Wineman 2009; Osowiecka 2016). To increase your potential for deeply benefiting from the practices in this journal, we offer the following suggestions:

- **Dedicate your space.** Cultivate a sense of reverence for the time and energy you are putting into your practice of writing. Choose a place to settle in that feels calming, grounding, and supportive for slowing down.

- **Set aside time.** Be intentional about the time you spend journaling. First, schedule a time each day that you will work on these exercises; marking your calendar with a daily practice increases the likelihood that you'll stay committed.

Second, consider setting a timer for ten to thirty minutes per response to help you stay focused on tuning in to your Wise Woman. Giving yourself a time limit helps prevent journaling from becoming overwhelming; it also provides a reminder to pause from the work you're doing and attend to the rest of your commitments between exercises.

- **Keep it personal.** If you're handwriting in this journal, select pens that feel comfortable to hold and ink colors that are pleasing to use. If you decide to type your responses on your computer, choose an enjoyable font or color to make your writing seem more personalized.

- **Go in any order.** You can skip around the exercises or go through them in order. Either approach is perfectly fine depending on what you prefer.

- **Go at your own pace.** Last, remember there is no wrong way to journal. Be gentle with yourself and take your time. You might return to certain prompts and skip others altogether. It's up to you.

You'll become acquainted with your Wise Woman and other magnificent parts of yourself, even if you've long forgotten them. You may be stretched out of your comfort zone from time to time, but this will increase your potential to achieve positive results!

Meet Your Guides

Debbie, your Peer Guide on this journey, is in recovery from BPD and complex post-traumatic stress disorder (cPTSD). She credits learning and practicing DBT skills with helping her embrace her emotional sensitivity and find balance, peace, and healing. She no longer meets the criteria for a BPD diagnosis and brings the wisdom of her personal transformation experience to each exercise. Debbie holds a bachelor of science degree in interdisciplinary studies (behavioral science, communication, and English) and a certificate in early childhood development; she has also completed professional-level DBT trainings. She teaches DBT skills as a peer educator online at DBT Path, a global psychoeducational school for emotionally sensitive people, and brings knowledge from this experience to the exercises in this journal as well.

Kathryn is a clinical social worker and trained in DBT while studying at Columbia University. She serves as your Professional Guide. Kathryn works with people who are learning to listen deeply to their inner wisdom, aka their Wise Woman, through honoring their emotions, listening to their bodies, and exploring how past experiences are informing the present. Her passion lies in helping others reclaim their most challenging experiences as sacred initiations for growing into their truest, wisest selves. She began studying DBT to combine her desire for body-mind-spirit integration with psychotherapy. In her private practice, Kathryn utilizes an approach that honors the full range of spiritual and emotional experiences and treats them as valid, important parts of life. She is currently pursuing her PhD in depth psychology with an emphasis in Jungian and archetypal studies to further this exploration of the psyche and soul.

Part 1

How to Listen to Your True Inner Voice

The foundation of building a life worth living is connecting to that sometimes subtle, sometimes not so subtle voice within ourselves. We call this inner voice our "Wise Woman." She is the part of us that knows and has access to something larger than our rational mind or emotional mind. She offers wisdom, insight, and deep knowing to every person on the planet. However, it's very easy to become disconnected and detached from this part of ourselves over time due to excess emotional stimulation, mistrust of our intuition and gut reactions, and a tendency to believe that all thoughts are facts.

In this journal, we offer mindfulness skills practice to help you become reacquainted with this part of yourself. Your Wise Woman has a powerful role to play in teaching you how to build a life that feels good, true, and satisfying. Mindfulness skills are designed to help you pay attention, on purpose, to one thing at a time. Noticing your thoughts, feeling your body from the inside out, and journaling practices are just a few of the mindful ways you can begin to slow down and listen to your Wise Woman. Part 1 offers a way to get to know her through experiential practice and exploration.

A Thought Is a Thesis

Goal:

* Practice noticing and challenging upsetting thoughts

Kathryn

One of the core skills for regulating our emotions and feeling more powerful in chaotic situations is learning how to notice our thoughts nonjudgmentally. While our thoughts are very persuasive when they occur to us, the adage "Thoughts aren't facts" can be a lifeline when we feel out of control. Thoughts are the by-product of our brains trying to protect us in our environment. Thoughts are *not* necessarily beacons of truth to obey at any cost, no matter how convincingly our emotions may lead us to believe otherwise. Knowing this distinction can give us freedom of choice. When we take our thoughts literally—*He hates me, I can't do it, I'll fail if I try*—we are locked into one reality. By practicing seeing our thoughts with flexibility and curiosity, we can begin to choose more realistic, even pleasurable thoughts that might serve us better in the long run.

While it's easy to say to yourself, "Thoughts aren't facts," in the heat of an emotional moment, it is much harder to make this distinction. People who are emotionally sensitive often need to learn tools to separate emotional thoughts from rational thoughts. One way to do this is to ask yourself the following questions:

* **Does my thought feel "charged" with emotion?** Meaning, is your thought coming from your emotional mind or your

Wise Woman? Usually when we feel a sense of indignation or martyrdom, or have trouble letting a thought go, there is some emotional component underneath our thinking. This is not wrong or bad but simply an indicator that we might need help seeing the situation from an outside and nonbiased perspective.

- **Would an objective observer (my therapist, friend, elementary-school teacher) agree with the "facts" I'm seeing?** Consider what other people would say are "facts." This is called "reality testing" and is a powerful way to check in with our own perception of a situation.

- **Is this thought familiar?** In other words, am I in a pattern of thinking that I often mistake as "fact"? This can be a pattern of self-loathing, self-victimization, or anger at the world and larger systems. Patterns of thinking can often sound like "facts" since we are so used to them. However, learning to identify a familiar pattern over what other people might consider "fact" is a helpful step in distinguishing thoughts from facts.

Debbie

In the past, I made many, many emotionally charged decisions triggered by inaccurate thoughts that were skewed by my previous experiences or current fears. I had to learn that just because I had a thought with an intense emotional reaction at the same time, it didn't mean that the thought was necessarily true. I learned to practice treating upsetting or dysregulating thoughts, regardless of how convincing, as theses to be proven or disproven before I took any action. With this approach, I began to reduce an immense amount of unnecessary suffering in my life.

You may also relate to sometimes taking your thoughts at face value. Sometimes they feel incredibly real and true because of your intense emotions. For example, you may have a distressing thought about a partner, such as, *He's going to leave me!* And, if this thought is accompanied by feeling terrified, you might become convinced that the thought is true—especially if people have left you in the past. The problem with this pattern is that you often end up experiencing unnecessary suffering and acting on undesired behaviors because you're reacting to thoughts that may *not* be true.

Exercise

Think about some upsetting thoughts you've had during the past week. For each:

List the distressing thought in one sentence (for example, "He's going to leave me").

_____

_____

List the accompanying intense feelings you have about this thought (for example, "Angry, sad, disappointed, ashamed, joyful, irritated").

_____

_____

_____

Ask yourself, *What are any irrefutable, solid facts that support this thought?* Think about observable facts that another reasonable person could also identify (rather than judgments, assumptions, fears, or other emotions). Also consider if any of the facts you identify feel charged with emotion or if they are recurring thought patterns. This can indicate that you need to keep going in terms of finding supportive, factual evidence for this thought. Write them down.

_____

_____

_____

_____

_____

_____

Now tune in to your Wise Woman. Ask her, "Is my distressing thought true? Are there facts that support its *opposite*?" (For example, "He's not going to leave me.") Write down these facts.

_____

_____

_____

_____

_____

_____

_____

What might a more balanced version of this thought sound like (for example, "I don't know if he's going to leave me")?

_____

_____

Tune in to your body: How does this middle-of-the-road thought feel? How might you skillfully respond to a similarly distressing thought in the future?

_____

_____

_____

_____

_____

_____

_____

_____

_____

_____

_____

_____

_____

Distressing thought: _____

_____

Intense feelings: _____

_____

Irrefutable, solid, observable facts that support this thought:

_____

_____

_____

_____

_____

_____

Is the distressing thought true? Are there facts that support its *opposite?*

_____

_____

_____

_____

_____

_____

_____

What might a more balanced version of this thought sound like?

_____

_____

How might you skillfully respond to a similarly distressing thought in the future?

_____

_____

_____

_____

_____

_____

_____

_____

_____

_____

_____

_____

_____

Distressing thought: _____

_____

Intense feelings: _____

_____

Irrefutable, solid, observable facts that support this thought:

_____

_____

_____

_____

_____

_____

Is the distressing thought true? Are there facts that support its *opposite?*

_____

_____

_____

_____

_____

_____

What might a more balanced version of this thought sound like?

_____

_____

How might you skillfully respond to a similarly distressing thought in the future?

_____

_____

_____

_____

_____

_____

_____

_____

_____

_____

_____

_____

_____

_____

Distressing thought: _____

_____

Intense feelings: _____

_____

Irrefutable, solid, observable facts that support this thought:

_____

_____

_____

_____

_____

_____

Is the distressing thought true? Are there facts that support its *opposite?*

_____

_____

_____

_____

_____

_____

What might a more balanced version of this thought sound like?

_____

_____

How might you skillfully respond to a similarly distressing thought in the future?

_____

_____

_____

_____

_____

_____

_____

_____

_____

_____

_____

_____

_____

_____

Distressing thought: _____

_____

Intense feelings: _____

_____

Irrefutable, solid, observable facts that support this thought:

_____

_____

_____

_____

_____

_____

Is the distressing thought true? Are there facts that support its *opposite?*

_____

_____

_____

_____

_____

_____

What might a more balanced version of this thought sound like?

_____

_____

How might you skillfully respond to a similarly distressing thought in the future?

_____

_____

_____

_____

_____

_____

_____

_____

_____

_____

_____

_____

_____

_____

_____

Accessing Your Inner Archetypes

Goals:

* Learn to trust your inner voice
* Practice working with your different states of mind: emotional, rational, and inner wisdom

Kathryn

In the beginning of this book we introduced the three states of mind characterized in DBT: emotional, rational, and inner wisdom (aka your Wise Woman). Now is a chance to delve more deeply into these. We all have a variety of inner characters. The cast can range from the "logical self" to the "emotional self," from the "fun self" to the "depressed self," and anything in between. These parts of our selves show up depending on where we are, whom we're around, and how we're feeling. They present themselves when we need new or different resources in a situation (for example, taking deep breaths to calm down, or knowing when to turn on upbeat music to shift your mood); at other times, they emerge out of habit (for example, someone not responding to a text message can automatically trigger your "anxious self").

The three main inner characters you'll be exploring in this chapter are your Wise, Emotional, and Rational Women. Your Emotional Woman is the part of you that feels deeply. She knows how to love and care, how to feel anger to protect, how to feel sadness to tend your wounds, and how to feel joy to celebrate the gifts of life. She has depth and dimension, and she adds texture to your world.

Your Rational Woman is a different animal. She is a thinker. She knows how to plan. She can get you from point A to point B on a project. She is like your inner computer: no feeling, only thinking. Without her, we would be in a soup of emotion without a map or structure. She is a vital component of being able to analyze a situation and think it through, step-by-step, and see multiple perspectives instead of reacting from emotions.

And finally, your Wise Woman. She is powerful. She's able to listen to your Emotional Woman and Rational Woman *at the same time.* She speaks through intuition, gut feeling, dreams, and deep knowing. She might even present options that have never occurred to you in your day-to-day habitual thinking and feeling patterns.

This practice is geared to help you get to know each of these women within you.

Debbie

I like this idea of having an internal support system that is working together for our best outcome. I have found that the key to finding balance with these various aspects of our selves is to first acknowledge that each part has an important role to play and that all are needed. For example, I used to become frustrated by and try to dismiss my Emotional Woman when I would become sensitive in response to someone's remarks. But I learned that her needs were as important as any other part of me. Through acknowledging and nurturing her by compassionately listening to her needs and underlying wisdom, instead of shutting her down, I began to heal many old wounds from my past.

With this example in mind, you can see how your Emotional Woman and Rational Woman would create an imbalance if either were solely at the forefront and giving no room to the other. Being guided exclusively by your emotional side can lead to irrational, emotionally driven choices that you later regret. Being driven only by reason or rationality neglects the important messages your emotions communicate, and it can create a disconnect between yourself and others. The goal is to have each of these parts of you meet in the middle, linked harmoniously and in balance by the wisdom of your Wise Woman.

Exercise

Let's explore each of these aspects of your self with curiosity. In the following exercise, without any self-censoring, and given the descriptions of the attributes of your Emotional Woman, Rational Woman, and Wise Woman, write out how you think each part of you would interpret and respond to recent situations that you found upsetting or dysregulating. Review the example and then add a couple of your own real-life situations. After you complete this assignment, write down your reflections. "Visualize Your Inner Archetypes." For a guided meditation that will help you visualize your Emotional, Rational, and Wise Woman, visit http://www.newharbinger.com /40613.

Example:

Situation: My significant other is running late for dinner plans and hasn't called.

Emotional Woman: He's being disrespectful! I'm getting angry. I feel scared! What if something happened to him? Maybe he's cheating on me!

Rational Woman: People run late sometimes. There's probably traffic at this hour. Maybe his cellphone battery died. This is not an emergency.

Wise Woman (synthesis of the responses of your Emotional and Rational Women)**:** It's normal for me to have some worry that a person I care about didn't show up when expected and hasn't called. I can wait, check the facts, and find out what happened, rather than become consumed by fear or jumping to conclusions.

Situation: _____

_____

_____

_____

Emotional Woman: _____

_____

_____

_____

Rational Woman: _____

_____

_____

_____

Wise Woman: _____

_____

_____

_____

_____

Reflection: _____

_____

_____

_____

_____

_____

Pleasurable Events Practice

Goal:

* ✸ Build a life that feels good by scheduling pleasure like it's your job

Kathryn

So often the moment people hear the word "pleasure," one of two things happens. They either lean in with curiosity and intrigue, or recoil with revulsion and disgust, as though pleasure is tainted, bad, wrong, and demoralizing. When we speak about pleasure in this journal, we are not talking about pleasure as some hedonistic free-for-all but rather as a practice of self-care that helps us build lives that feel satisfying daily, even when life gets hard.

Pleasure is also, as is the case with the simple gifts in life, not something that always comes easily. It takes practice, since so many of us have learned how to live in a *stress response* (a behavioral state focused on protecting ourselves from danger). The key is to work on orienting toward what feels nourishing and satisfying in life.

The point of practicing pleasure day to day is to help build a foundation for emotional resiliency. It's way easier to manage the challenges of life when we have a baseline of feeling at ease and grounded. As emotionally sensitive people, it's as though our emotional sensors (I picture these as antennae that run throughout our bodies and nervous systems) are on high alert. These antennae pick up *everything*—the good, bad, and ugly. And because they're so sensitive, they need lots of care so they don't burn out.

As an emotionally sensitive person, you are at risk for your antennae to go haywire and pick up all kinds of information—like a scrambled TV set—which can leave you in lots of emotional distress. You can think of practicing pleasure as caring for the valuable, intuitive antennae connected to your Wise Woman.

Debbie

I love the imagery of antennae that run through our sensory systems and help us pick up on the world around us. I can relate to becoming overwhelmed and feeling frazzled when I haven't prioritized my self-care or taken time to slow down, rest, and restore. I must take action at that point to prevent emotional dysregulation. One of my favorite ways of recalibrating my sensors is to take a relaxing, mindful shower using really nice body washes with scents—jasmine, lavender, or coconut—that help soothe me. Instead of rushing through the process, I set time aside to enjoy each moment. I feel the warmth of the water, smell the delicious scents, and lovingly care for myself by putting on lotion or body butter afterward. I plan ahead to carve out the time to do this so that I don't feel rushed.

Practicing self-care helps relieve stress and trains your body and mind to become more resilient when faced with future stressful situations. Could you imagine taking some time to do something like this for yourself? Maybe you're out of practice with doing fun or pleasurable things. Whether you've had a long run of depression, have been busy de-prioritizing yourself beneath a million tasks and other people, or you've come to believe that you are unworthy of (or don't have time to) take care of yourself in this way (and I've certainly experienced all of the above!), we've got some work to do. Some fun work. I promise.

Exercise

What are some activities that you enjoy? These can be simple things like spending time with your pet, dancing, baking, or going for walks. If there's a lack of pleasurable activities in your life right now, what are some things you used to find joy in that you may be able to revisit and rekindle? A love for being in nature? Singing? Artwork? Reading? Writing?

Make a list and set an intention that you'll practice at least one pleasurable activity from your list this week. Again, this is a practice, and it can take your body and emotions some time to open up and feel pleasure if you are used to being stressed, depressed, or on edge. Write down what you notice after practicing pleasure. "Soothe Your Inner Antennae." For a guided meditation to help you self-soothe, visit http://www.newharbinger.com/40613.

_____

_____

_____

_____

_____

_____

_____

_____

_____

_____

_____

_____

Who Is Running the Show in a Crisis?

Goal:

* Identify the parts of yourself that take over in a crisis

Kathryn

Sometimes, despite our best attempts and most heartfelt efforts, a crisis gets the best of us—and we end up making a bad situation worse. In these moments, it can feel as though we are being "hijacked" by a part of ourselves that feels out of control and desperate to feel better. When emotionally sensitive people don't know how to cope effectively in stressful situations, we resort to behaviors that aren't in alignment with our highest self and long-term goals. We know we are in the grip of desperation when, after the crisis, we wonder why in the world we said that thing or did that other thing or felt so "beside ourselves."

This practice is intended to help you listen to the part of yourself that you resort to in a crisis. You will explore your deeper needs and hear from your Wise Woman, who has effectively coped in a crisis in the past, to see if she has any tips for you.

Debbie

At one point in my life I believed that my parents' only saving grace was that they didn't know any better when they were raising me. My parents were young, broken people who were raised by young, broken people. They did the best they could with very limited parenting skills. Does this sound familiar? Perhaps you were raised in a less than ideal home environment and inherited dysfunctional coping patterns by observing your caretakers. Extending compassion to them in retrospect (and to you in the present) can be tremendously challenging, but doing so can help you understand the motivations of the part of you that emerges in a crisis.

Now *you* are the one doing the best you can. When you're feeling overwhelmed or triggered, it is likely that, instead of your Wise Woman, another part of you initially shows up to be acknowledged. This is the part that may have been hurt in the past or experienced trauma. She's still there, and she wears the cloak of being in crisis mode.

I love the idea of taking some time to validate the wounded parts of yourself. With practice, your Wise Woman can become a source of comfort and care when doing this important work. During this exercise, be careful to notice any judgments you make when you reflect on a past situation that might still be painful. Remember that your Wise Woman in crisis mode wasn't acting out to deliberately hurt you. She was trying to get her needs met. She was in pain and needed help. This exercise offers an opportunity to lovingly re-parent, reassure, and redirect her now.

Exercise

To begin, consider a time when you didn't cope as well as you had hoped. Maybe it was after a long day at work or at a stressful family event. Think about where you were, what you were feeling, and what your day had been like leading up to this experience. See yourself as though you are in a movie noticing all the different scenes and scenarios. When you are ready, begin journaling from the perspective of your emotional mind. This is the part of you that perhaps became overwhelmed, scared, or lost in this scene. What did you need that you didn't get? What was going on around you that felt so overwhelming or difficult? Use a compassionate ear to really listen to this part of yourself as you write.

_____

_____

_____

_____

_____

_____

_____

_____

_____

_____

_____

_____

_____

_____

_____

_____

When you have finished writing, change perspectives. Consider the same situation from the perspective of your Wise Woman. What does this part of you see, and what would she have done to not make this stressful situation worse? How would she have acted? Felt? Done? Write from the voice of your Wise Woman who knows how to self-parent and take care of you well.

_____

_____

_____

_____

_____

_____

_____

_____

_____

_____

_____

_____

_____

_____

_____

_____

Open and Listen to Your Heart

Goal:

* Increase awareness of physical sensation through movement

Kathryn

Mindfulness practices are the heart of DBT skills, yet they often get overlooked because they are also some of the most challenging! Mindfulness often rings of boring, bland, and agitating practices that can be a major hurdle for people whose minds and emotions are strong and active. Instead of sitting still, this mindfulness *movement* can be a powerful practice to help you reconnect with your inner wisdom and felt sensations without getting lost in overwhelming feelings. We don't want you to avoid mindfulness skills altogether due to fear of boredom or lack of interest!

This practice is intended to help you move from your head—where so many of us live—into your heart—where many people experience their Wise Woman. In this exercise, you'll literally *feel* your heart so that you can tap into the wisdom it wishes to convey. Like yoga, this exercise will help you link feeling, breath, and movement. It will end with a journaling prompt.

Debbie

My yoga instructor often reminds students to practice "living below the neck." Kathryn mentioned how, like yoga, this exercise encourages you to be in your heart, mindfully aware of your breath, feelings, and movements. As an emotionally sensitive person, your body awareness is likely often focused above the neck and in your mind with lots of worrying and trying to figure out ways to feel better. Because of this, you have probably become oblivious to sensation-based signals and feelings that are speaking to you from other parts of your body. I can certainly relate! Yoga and exercises like the one outlined in this chapter have been instrumental in helping me become more aware of the rest of my body, allowing me to tap into my body's messages of wisdom.

In this exercise, you get to take some time to move your attention down from your thinking, planning, reasoning mind to a sensation-based activity in your heart. You get to slow down enough to notice the amazingness of it beating in your chest, something we all take for granted and that naturally fades into the background of our awareness from day to day. And you get to approach your heart symbolically as a source of wisdom, a part of you that has a voice that can be heard if you listen hard enough to its whispers. What is your heart telling you today?

Exercise

Begin by gently closing your eyes and bringing attention to the feeling of your heart in your chest. If needed, gently place your hand on your chest and notice if you can physically feel your heartbeat. Take three long breaths here. With each breath, notice if you can let your mind travel to your heart, as though with each breath you shift deeper from your head to your heart. "Guided Heart Opening Practice." For a guided practice to help you open your heart, visit http://www .newharbinger.com/40613.

Continuing to breathe gently and deeply, and begin to gently stretch your chest by opening the front of your body. Allow your shoulder blades to get close enough to lightly kiss one another. Then, on your exhale, allow the back of your heart to open by curling forward, hunching your shoulders gently toward one another. Then repeat—opening gently to the front and then to the back. Repeat three times.

Now, returning to your journal, feel the sensation of your physical heart. What do you notice? How does your heart feel today? What does your heart have to say today? Note any feelings, words, or images that come forward after connecting with your body consciously. With this exercise, "following your heart" becomes a practice that is more connected, clear, and grounded than you could ever imagine.

_____

_____

_____

_____

_____

_____

_____

_____

_____

Handling Life Stress, Upsets, and Triggers

This part of the journal will encourage you to shift from *reacting* to *responding* when you're feeling emotionally triggered. We'll look at *distress tolerance* skills, which are also considered "crisis survival" skills. Emotionally sensitive people often have difficulty tolerating situations that have no immediate remedy or solution, especially if they are experiencing emotional pain. The tendency is to act on impulsive urges, often making the original triggering situation worse.

Part 2 is about slowing down in challenging moments. You'll use mindfulness skills to be aware of your emotional experiences and urges, and to prepare to respond more skillfully to future triggering events. In addition, you'll have opportunities to nonjudgmentally reflect on past behaviors that you regret so that you can better understand what led to those choices and make different ones in the future.

Plan Ahead to Feel Better in the Moment

Goal:

* Plan ahead for predictably challenging or stressful situations by imagining a real scenario

Kathryn

A Wise Woman (my mom) once said, "A predictable problem is a preventable problem." While this might not *always* be true, it sure does help to plan ahead for emotionally challenging situations. Sometimes you might avoid thinking about future events because you know they are going to be challenging—and you don't want to suffer in advance in addition to being distressed during the actual event. The feeling you're avoiding is called *anticipatory anxiety.*

It's good self-care practice to plan ahead for your personal challenges instead of trying to white-knuckle it when the time comes. This journaling exercise is intended to help you consider an upcoming stressful event—maybe it's getting home after a long day, going to a meeting at work, driving in dense traffic, or going to a family event. This preparation is like a dress rehearsal for the neurons in your brain. Visualizing a situation and planning ahead for it can help you feel prepared and more at ease when you're in the actual moment.

Debbie

This skillful act of planning ahead for stressful events can help you learn how to get through situations that until now have seemed impossible. I know firsthand. Things that I avoided because they were so anxiety provoking, like getting dental work or going to a routine OB-GYN appointment (for fear of becoming triggered and inconsolably dysregulated), became doable.

As I mention in a more in-depth look at this skill in my book, *Stronger Than BPD*, planning ahead is the same practice that professional athletes use when they prepare for success in a big game or competition. They use their imaginations to visualize the event in advance, vividly anticipating every nuance they can; they envision themselves succeeding.

You're doing the same thing with this exercise. Instead of allowing fear and anxiety to write the ending of the story, your Wise Woman will come forth with an alternate ending, one in which you are successfully coping with your anxiety-provoking circumstances.

Exercise

"Visualize Coping Well." For a guided visualization practice of coping well, visit http://www.newharbinger.com/40613. Consider a future event that is causing you some distress and that you may be tempted to avoid thinking about. Begin by writing about this situation from your perspective in present tense (using "I am" rather than "I will"). What is going on around you? Where are you? Who is with you? What is your role in this situation? How do you feel?

Be specific and detailed. Here is how your journal entry might start:

I just got home. I've had a long day at work. I feel alone and stressed, but I don't know what to do. I feel anxious. No one is home with me. I don't want to make my night a "bad night," but I don't know what else to do...

_____

_____

_____

_____

_____

_____

_____

_____

_____

_____

_____

_____

_____

_____

_____

_____

_____

_____

After considering the predictable situation, call upon your Wise Woman. Imagine yourself tapping into the well of resources that your Wise Woman possesses and that you've used to get through challenges in the past. What would your future situation look like if your Wise Woman were running the show? Would she do anything differently than what you're used to doing?

_____

_____

_____

_____

_____

_____

_____

_____

_____

_____

_____

_____

_____

_____

_____

When you have finished viewing this situation from the perspective of your Wise Woman, identify three to five things you can do to prepare for this upcoming experience.

1. _____

_____

_____

2. _____

_____

_____

3. _____

_____

_____

4. _____

_____

_____

5. _____

_____

_____

Your Superpowers

* Draw on new or hard-to-remember inner
   resources

Kathryn

Living in a world that so often tells us that we need to be better,
stronger, faster, thinner, and so on makes it hard to see and appreciate our superpowers. Particularly with emotionally sensitive people, it
can be difficult to even imagine that our greatest challenge (feeling
the world deeply) could also be our greatest strength.

This exercise is focused on helping you identify your superpowers
through the blessing of *projection*. Projection is a psychological
defense mechanism by which we attribute our own traits, whether
"good" or "bad," to other people. Put another way, sometimes we see
our most valuable gifts in *other* people.

Debbie

Years ago, I was hooked on a cheesy TV show called *Drop Dead Diva*.
The main character, Jane, is a plus-size attorney (who in a previous
life was a thin fashion model), and she carries herself with confidence, calling upon her intelligence and acceptance of her new body
and new beauty. When I have struggled with self-confidence or
feeling inferior, I have thought about how I also have the superpower

of self-confidence within. Using this example, my exercise looks something like this:

"I am like Jane [admirable person/character] because I also possess self-confidence [superpower/inner resource] and this is how I show it: I watch my posture so that I am not slouched. I give eye contact. I speak my mind and get my needs met."

I have also plugged in Scully from *The X-Files* (for her superpowers of objectivity, skepticism, calmness, and professionalism) and Lorelai from *Gilmore Girls* (for her quick-thinking wit, easy-going nature, and sense of humor).

Give this exercise a try, and have fun with it!

Exercise

Consider someone you admire. This person could be real or fictional.

Let your imagination roll. If this person is real, what is it about him that you honor? What does he seem to possess that you don't? If this character is imaginary what is her superpower? Where did it come from and how did she learn to use it? Choose one person or character and write out a full description of his or her strengths, weaknesses, resources, and challenges. You could even draw a picture of him or her if you desire.

_____

_____

_____

_____

_____

_____

_____

_____

_____

_____

_____

_____

_____

_____

_____

_____

_____

_____

_____

Next, explore how you already demonstrate this character's super-power in your own life. How have you shown, or currently show, these traits—resilience, strength, grace, patience, or whatever it is that you find admirable—in your own life? If you need prompting, complete this sentence:

I am like _____ [admirable person/character]

because I also possess _____

_____ [superpower/inner resource]

and this is how I show it: _____

_____

_____

_____

_____

_____

_____

_____

_____

_____

_____

_____

Consider this your own hidden superpower and notice how and when you use it. Often when we make unconscious resources conscious, they start to show their power and magic, so prepare to be surprised at your own resourcefulness.

Mental Health Vacation

Goal:

* Use imagination (imagery) to improve
  the moment

Kathryn

In DBT, imagery is a tool for improving stressful moments through taking a "mental vacation" and imagining a place that helps you feel calmer or more at ease. The following exercise is designed to help you practice turning your mind toward a more relaxing mental space, rather than staying stuck in the familiar places of chaos and crisis.

Imagine this: You're in the midst of a very stressful situation. You suddenly realize there is nothing you can do to fix it in this moment. So you decide to just drop everything, jump on a plane, and head to a tropical destination. Feels great to imagine escaping, right?

Of course, running away would be avoiding your problem, and most of the time it's unrealistic anyway. You're busy living your life and need to stick around to work through your issues, yet you desperately need a break. So allow yourself one! Keep in mind that self-care doesn't have to be time consuming or elaborate. This skill is one you can use anytime and anywhere to help you feel rejuvenated.

Debbie

It may feel counterintuitive to step away from an unresolved stressful situation temporarily, but in small doses this may be the most skillful thing to do. When you're distressed, realizing that problem-solving isn't getting you anywhere, and you don't want to make matters worse, temporary distraction can be incredibly helpful for regulating intense emotions.

In this exercise, you'll harness the power of your vivid imagination. You might be aware that you frequently use your imagination in ways that create unnecessary suffering, such as projecting into a fearful future of catastrophic possibilities. But, in this exercise, you'll be empowering yourself to improve your overall sense of well-being by channeling that creative energy in a positive way. This time-limited activity is about choosing to create a mini mental hiatus from your stress without completely avoiding it.

Exercise

"Taking a Mental Health Vacation." For a guided meditation to help you access an inner vacation, visit http://www.newharbinger.com /40613. Find a quiet space that smells nice and has dim lighting. Turn off your electronic devices. Set a timer for fifteen minutes. Close your eyes and begin to envision your ideal vacation. What destination have you chosen? What season is it? What is the weather like? What time of day is it? Are you alone, or did you to choose bring other people or animals? Did you bring any belongings? What do you hear, smell, see, feel, and taste? What do you feel like doing in this special place? Spend these fifteen minutes soaking up this vacation.

Once you've completed your mental health vacation, journal what you can remember about your experience and how you feel. Refer to this visualization in the future when you need another mental break.

Acknowledging When Life Goes Right

Goal:

* ✸ Use comparisons and a gratitude list to increase positive feelings

Kathryn

During life challenges or when learning how to manage overwhelming emotions, sometimes we might feel as if life is simply the worst. As emotionally sensitive people, it might feel challenging to move out of painful emotions and experiences, yet in DBT we practice skills that help us learn to appreciate the full spectrum of life—the painful all the way to the nourishing and satisfying. Learning how to appreciate life even in the most frustrating circumstances can take practice, and using comparisons and gratitude is one tool to try.

In DBT, we are asked to notice the many aspects of our life experiences, not only the challenging parts. This helps retrain the brain and body to pick up information that is nourishing, no matter how small (a smile from a stranger, an email from a friend, a good meal) rather than focusing on only what's going wrong. This is important, because we can get so used to anticipating disaster that we overlook pleasure and satisfaction, which are healing and relaxing to the body and soul.

This exercise is a practice you can use to help refocus your mind and body to begin savoring the satisfying parts of your life. This doesn't mean you ignore the painful and challenging ones. Rather, you're learning how to appreciate and honor your whole life experience. The activity can help you consider the underlying gifts of your life, despite how painful life can be sometimes, particularly when you make a habit of it.

Debbie

I know from experience that when you're emotionally sensitive, comparing yourself to those less fortunate can trigger intense emotions and be a recipe for emotional dysregulation. If someone were to remind me of the struggles of starving children in Africa when I express a first world problem (for example, the pizza delivery guy forgot the crushed pepper!), I might feel not only shame at having complained about something so petty, but I'd feel bad for the children in Africa too! But that's not the intention of this practice. The skill of comparing our lives to those who are less fortunate isn't about feeling better because someone else has it worse. It's about feeling grateful that it could be worse for us, and it isn't.

For example, at the moment, I'm single. In fact, I've been single for a while. Sometimes I feel lonely, which can lead to sadness and thoughts of whether I'll ever find my true companion. In these moments, I can use the skill of *comparisons* to remember a time when being alone felt even worse, when it was intolerable and would cause me to spiral into a crisis. Or I can recall when I was in an unhealthy relationship that made me feel even lonelier because I wasn't seen and appreciated. Now when I feel lonely, I know that I can seek out connection through friends, going to a yoga class, or calling a loved one. I can also tolerate the feeling of loneliness and know that it will pass. Comparing where I am now to where I was before with BPD helps regulate my mood and reminds me that things could be worse— but they aren't.

Exercise

Now it's your turn. For this journaling exercise, practice savoring the gifts of life. Below are prompts to help you get started. You could make a list, write a letter, or simply journal your responses.

What things are going well in your life?

What are you grateful for?

Compare and contrast your situation with someone who has it worse, or compare and contrast how you are better able to cope today than you may have in the past.

_____

_____

_____

_____

_____

_____

_____

_____

_____

_____

_____

_____

_____

_____

_____

_____

_____

_____

Note how you feel after you complete this exercise.

_____

_____

_____

_____

_____

_____

_____

_____

_____

_____

_____

Get Out of Your Mind

Goal:

* Elicit positive feelings by getting outside of yourself and helping others

Kathryn

A surefire way to feel better about yourself and about life in general is to help someone else. It can be easy to get stuck in your own mind and with your own life concerns. An antidote to this is to step into someone else's shoes and be of service. While noticing thoughts and feelings are essential skills in self-awareness and emotion regulation, the feeling of *interconnection* can be a powerful resource when you are caught in your own mental narrative or experiencing challenging emotions.

Being of service to someone else does not require becoming Mother Theresa or Gandhi. The skill is simply to take action (rather than thinking about it) to support another person. The action you choose can be as large or as small as you desire—a kind note on a coworker's desk, a candy bar left in a friend's mailbox, or even a phone call to ask about volunteering at a local organization. The size of the action is much less important than your intention behind it, which, for DBT purposes, is to help build positive emotional experiences.

Often people ask, "But isn't it selfish to give to others so I feel better?" For this skill, we are putting that question to the test. You are encouraged to consider whether helping someone helps you feel positive feelings and if this might prompt you to do more.

Debbie

When we're dysregulated emotionally, we're susceptible to entering a vortex of fear and self-absorption. And when we're in the vortex, we're not aware of any other parts of our experience. There was a time in my life when I was so consumed by my own problems, worries, and concerns that I barely noticed that there were other things going on in the world around me. If you can relate to this, it may seem very counterintuitive in such moments to consider stepping outside of your own experience to help someone else, but I've found that setting aside preoccupation with my problems and concerns is an effective way to take a break from the madness and gain some emotional equilibrium.

Exercise

Here are some ways that you can practice being a support to others:

- Call a lonely elderly relative

- Send someone a surprise greeting card in the mail

- Pay for someone's lunch

- Gather up some items you're not using anymore and donate them to the local thrift store

- Create care packages for the homeless

- Deliver pet food to an animal shelter

What are some things you are willing to try to step out of your own experience temporarily and serve others?

List them here, leaving some space between each so you can update this journal entry with the dates you completed the tasks and how you felt afterward. Come back to this list when you're in need of ideas for getting out of your mind.

Part 3

Strengthening Your Emotional Resiliency from the Inside Out

No doubt, you've noticed that when you're not feeling well physically—be it a cold, headache, PMS, or because you've had a blood sugar drop from waiting too long to eat—your emotional state is impacted. You might have noticed that during such times you're moody, more irritable, and become angry more quickly. It's not your imagination, and it happens to everyone. When our bodies are focused on restoring physical equilibrium due to illness, hunger, or hormonal changes it can be more challenging to be emotionally balanced. That's why it's so important not to minimize the power of your mind-body connection. Bottom line: taking care of your physical health is essential to your emotional well-being, and the skills in part 3 are crucial for feeling emotionally stable.

Being emotionally sensitive means that you might feel the impact of physical imbalance on your emotional health more strongly than others. On top of that, when you're predisposed biologically, environmentally, or culturally to emotional sensitivity, knowing how to lovingly and consistently care for yourself may not come naturally. In this case, it takes your willingness to explore and practice various skills to discover what helps you feel strong and stable. The good news is that this is completely possible to do!

In this section of the journal, you'll work through prompts designed to help you increase your emotional resiliency and decrease emotional vulnerability by paying attention to your mind-body connection. You'll explore nurturing activities focused on taking care of your physical health. You'll learn how to connect with and stay better attuned to your Wise Woman, who can easily be forgotten when you're stressing, worrying, or having intense emotional experiences. She can be a powerful ally in finding a healthy balance of physical and emotional self-care.

Being Mindful of Your Body

Goals:

* Listen to your Wise Woman by feeling your body from the inside out

* Pay attention to physical cues and signals to engage in self-care effectively

* Learn to heed signals from your Wise Woman, including cues for hunger, fullness, tiredness, and energy level

Kathryn

Through the course of a busy day or in the midst of challenging life circumstances, it's easy to become detached from our bodies. Part of feeling burned out is due to ignoring the signals our bodies are giving us instead of paying attention to our feelings and taking compassionate action to meet our needs. In DBT, emotion regulation is less about crisis management techniques and more about developing consistent life skills that help us build a foundation of emotional health. Being in tune with our bodies sets this foundation for internal emotional stability.

To build emotional health and resiliency that can withstand the challenging parts of life (no matter how large or small), connecting to your body and listening to what you need is a crucial skill. Being able to notice when your body is hungry, tired, longing for connection, or satisfied is part of a strong self-care practice. Your Wise Woman can guide you in taking care of *you*. When you practice tuning in to the needs of your Wise Woman and begin listening to her signals, you're already on your way to greater emotional stability.

Debbie

It's true that emotion regulation skills are designed to help you create a balanced, healthy, more resilient lifestyle so that you can handle life's ups and downs more effectively. If you're learning these skills while experiencing certain intense emotions on a regular basis, you may need some extra support to build that balance.

When someone is feeling intense sadness or anxiety, the internal sensors that cue him or her to feelings of hunger and fullness may be out of whack and hard to discern. If this is true for you, you may not be aware of the signals your body is sending you and end up skipping meals or overeating. I know this to be true. In the past, I struggled with anxiety symptoms that were so severe that I wouldn't experience the physical sensation of hunger for days on end. I worked with a psychiatric nurse to come up with an eating plan (more like an eating schedule) to be sure that, whether I felt hungry or not, I was eating to keep my blood sugar balanced so I would feel strong of mind and body. For other people, it may be harder to feel fullness and satisfaction, which may lead to overeating and mistrust of hunger signals. Either end of the spectrum is unhealthy for the body and mind, and can cause us to have mood swings, trouble focusing, or to feel unbalanced emotionally.

If your hunger sensors are difficult to detect, it's essential that you check in with your physician or psychiatrist to figure out how to best care for yourself to get them back on track. The exercise that follows is a good starting point for slowing down and noticing what's happening in your body so that you can have that conversation with yourself. (You can download a guided meditation of this exercise called "Sensing Your Body Practice" at http://www.newharbinger

.com/40613.) Even if you're not experiencing a total absence of hunger and/or fullness cues, practicing mindfully checking in with your body to gauge your hunger and energy levels can be helpful for forming and maintaining healthy eating habits. Give this exercise a try at random times throughout the day, and log your results to help you increase awareness of your physical cues.

Exercise

Begin by taking three deep breaths. Allow yourself to slow down as you begin this exercise.

As you settle into your breathing, take an inventory of the following feelings and journal your responses below:

What is your hunger level right now on a scale of 1 to 10 (10 being most hungry)?

_____

If your hunger is between 3 and 5, do you want a snack? If so, what would it be? Why?

_____

_____

_____

_____

_____

_____

If your hunger is between 5 and 8, do you want a meal? If so, what do you want to eat? Why?

_____

_____

_____

_____

_____

_____

If your hunger is above an 8, what do you need to eat to satisfy yourself? Why?

_____

_____

_____

_____

_____

_____

What is your energy level right now, on a scale of 1 to 10?

_____

If your energy level is under a 5, do you need to rest and restore? How?

_____

_____

_____

_____

_____

_____

If your energy level is above a 5, do you need to release some energy? How?

_____

_____

_____

_____

_____

_____

_____

Based on this information, ask your Wise Woman, "What do you need today?" Notice if she is longing for connection, time in nature to decompress, a funny book to read, or something else. Let this last prompt be intuitive—trust what you sense.

_____

_____

_____

_____

_____

_____

_____

_____

_____

_____

_____

_____

_____

_____

_____

_____

_____

Your Off-Screen Performance

Goal:

* Develop an evening ritual of creating a space to write and engaging in self-care

Kathryn

In a study on the impact of sleep, researchers explored sleep deprivation and our ability to recognize emotional facial cues (Maccari et al. 2014). What they found was that people who were sleep deprived were less able to recognize neutral facial expressions than when they had adequate sleep. Furthermore, research also suggests that sleep and emotional processing are highly linked and impact one another (Deliens, Gilson, and Peigneux 2014). What this means is that getting enough good-quality sleep is vital to being emotionally effective at knowing what we and others are feeling. This is especially important to consider for people who are naturally emotionally sensitive. It's no wonder that DBT classifies getting regular, balanced sleep as a primary emotion regulation skill.

Yet getting a good night's rest might seem like a distant fantasy if sleep is a struggle. Rumination, excess emotional energy, and worry thoughts are all factors that can impact our ability to relax into sleep. Often people need more lead time than simply hopping into bed to help the body transition from wakefulness to sleep.

Developing a nighttime ritual is one way to support your body, mind, and emotions to prepare for sleep so that going to bed isn't something you dread. This exercise is focused on helping you explore your natural nightly routine and evaluate its effectiveness in helping you sleep. You'll also create a new evening ritual so that you can get a nourishing night's rest.

Debbie

Sleep deprivation, combined with emotional sensitivity, is a surefire recipe for feeling unbalanced and emotionally dysregulated during the day. A lack of sleep can lead to unnecessary misunderstandings or arguments (because you're irritable), avoidable mistakes (because you're unfocused), and other upsetting mishaps.

I once showed up at work barely able to keep my eyes open, feeling on edge, irritable, and anxious after getting only two hours of sleep. I'd been stressing out about a meeting coming up in the morning, and instead of doing something relaxing before bed, I worked on spreadsheets and scrolled through online news and social media until I finally passed out from exhaustion. The next day at work, I could barely focus in the meeting and felt grouchy and out of it all day. I wasn't feeling confident, prepared, or professional—getting inadequate sleep meant I didn't set myself up for success. This was not an isolated incident, and unhealthy habits like this were clearly reducing my emotional resiliency. I needed to make some changes to my routine.

Can you relate? Do you have trouble getting regular, restful, restorative sleep? Do you often feel tired in the morning or as if you're dragging your feet all day? The good news is that there are things you can do to help you get the rest you desperately want and need.

Exercise

Think about your evening routine and sleep habits. Then answer the following questions:

What do you typically do right before going to bed? Do you stay up until the last minute watching television or browsing the Internet? Eat? Worry about the next day?

_____

_____

_____

_____

_____

_____

_____

_____

_____

_____

_____

_____

_____

_____

What do you find to be a challenge at night? Is it going to sleep? Relaxing after work? Dealing with anxiety that comes up? Engaging in unhealthy habits (substance abuse, emotional eating, arguing)?

_____

_____

_____

_____

_____

_____

_____

What would an ideal, nourishing evening look like to you? What would you be doing? Who would be present? What time would you start winding down, and what time would you actually want to be asleep?

_____

_____

_____

_____

_____

_____

_____

_____

List the ways you want to improve your nightly routine. For example:

- Not watching the news or an emotionally charged show right before bed (so that you're not getting triggered and activating your nervous system when you want to be winding down).

- Shutting down electronic devices two hours before sleep time (because light from devices can inhibit your body's production of melatonin, a natural sleep-inducing hormone; also, interesting stories and videos will keep you up).

- Engaging in a short breathing or meditation practice to calm and relax your body and mind.

- Releasing lingering worries by visualizing putting those issues on hold until the next day.

_____

_____

_____

_____

_____

_____

_____

_____

_____

_____

As you begin trying various new ways of approaching your evening routine, make notes about what you notice the next morning. For example, did not watching television before bed or watching a neutral or nonemotionally charged show seem to impact your sleep in a positive way? Did you have an easier time drifting off to sleep on nights when you're shutting down electronic devices a couple of hours before you'd like to be asleep? Return to this journal entry and update any differences you notice because of taking better care of yourself in the evening.

_____

_____

_____

_____

_____

_____

_____

_____

_____

_____

_____

_____

_____

_____

_____

_____

_____

_____

_____

_____

_____

_____

_____

_____

_____

_____

_____

_____

_____

_____

_____

_____

_____

_____

_____

_____

_____

_____

_____

Self-Care Using Your Senses
Caring for Your Wise Woman

Goals:

* Develop a practice of self-care and self-love

* Practice being gentle to and compassionate with yourself by using self-soothing skills

* Move from self-punishment to self-care to prevent shame and self-loathing

Kathryn

One of my favorite skills to practice and to teach is *self-soothing*, which is when you calm your nervous system by activating one of your five senses (touch, taste, sound, sight, smell). Comforting yourself is something that many people must learn as adults due to growing up in homes and environments that didn't demonstrate how to be gentle and understanding.

Habitual patterns of self-punishment and self-judgment add distress to your life. You can counter these negative habits by learning how to self-soothe. It's an important tool to have in your pocket for whenever you notice that your stress levels are increasing or when you're feeling judgmental of your emotions, decisions, or needs. Self-soothing might feel unfamiliar at first, but, with practice, you can learn to treat yourself with gentleness and care instead of criticism.

Learning how to shift to self-care from self-punishment begins with taking the compassionate stance that you deserve care and soothing when in distress. Self-soothing will help you build *self-trust*, which is a belief that you can handle life and its challenges because you know how to take care of yourself. This underlying feeling that you are you own best caretaker is powerful in supporting your emotional health and resiliency, and it takes practice to develop this kind of relationship with yourself.

Debbie

Do you remember soothing yourself as a child? When I was six, I had difficulty managing my emotions whenever Nana (my grandmother) would end a visit. I'd cry and become inconsolable…until Nana gave me a doll that she said I could pretend was her. I could hug "Nana Baby" whenever Nana was away. You know what? It worked! I would hold and kiss that doll and tell her all the things I would've told my Nana had she been there in those moments. I felt so comforted and able to handle those once-dreaded separations. I was self-soothing with a doll!

Although I had this positive experience of self-soothing in childhood, as an adult I found it counterintuitive when my therapist suggested that I do nurturing and comforting things for myself in times of distress. I figured it wouldn't solve my problems, so what was the point? It seemed a waste of time and shameful for me to, for example, choose to cuddle up on the couch and watch a movie when I was stressing about a friend having a serious operation in the morning. *How dare I enjoy myself during this serious, upsetting, horrible time?* I would think. *How selfish that would be of me!*

The truth is, self-soothing won't solve our problems—it's not meant to. It didn't bring my grandmother back to our house any sooner, and it wouldn't cause my friend to not need an operation. But the act of self-care through self-soothing isn't selfish. That's a big misconception. Self-soothing can help you reduce suffering in difficult moments. By allowing your nervous system to relax and by providing a much-needed break from upsetting circumstances, you can prevent yourself from spiraling into further emotional dysregulation. I now use self-soothing regularly and highly recommend it to anyone who'll listen. Please give it a try. My guess is that you will not regret it, and you'll have a tool that you can truly feel good about using to take better care of yourself.

Exercise

This prompt will help you identify what self-soothing might look like for you and how to begin caring for yourself.

Start by creating an atmosphere of calm and comfort. This could entail lighting a candle, snuggling up in a cozy blanket, or making yourself a cup of tea. Once you're comfortable, answer the following questions:

What is your habitual response to stress or emotional pain?

Do you fall into self-judgment and blame? What does this feel like?

Do you find yourself being self-critical? What do you say to yourself in these moments?

Do you shut down? If so, what triggers this?

Are you gentle with yourself? How does this feel?

_____

_____

_____

_____

_____

_____

_____

_____

_____

_____

_____

_____

_____

_____

_____

_____

_____

_____

_____

_____

_____

_____

Self-Care Using Your Senses

What does your Wise Woman know about self-care? What does she need when you are in emotional pain?

_____

_____

_____

_____

_____

_____

_____

_____

_____

_____

_____

_____

_____

_____

_____

_____

_____

Write down three ways you can practice self-care for your *body* (for example, giving a self-massage, taking a warm bath, taking a walk, cooking a good meal, putting your bare feet on the grass):

_____

_____

_____

_____

Write down three ways you can practice self-care for your *mind* (for example, watching a funny movie, talking with a friend, looking out the window at the trees, doing a crossword puzzle):

_____

_____

_____

_____

Write down three ways you can practice self-care for your *soul* (for example, reading a meaningful book; meditating, praying, or contemplating; connecting with a pet):

_____

_____

_____

_____

Practice at least one of the ideas you came up with as a way of putting self-love into action. Afterward, take some time to write how it went.

How did you feel using your self-care skills? What felt nourishing and what felt challenging? Keep practicing, and this will become easier with time.

_____

_____

_____

_____

_____

_____

_____

_____

_____

_____

_____

_____

_____

_____

_____

_____

_____

Walk This Way (Mindfully)

Goals:

* Practice being in the present moment in a familiar place

* Allow your Wise Woman to lead you into presence

Kathryn

Another key skill in DBT is learning how to pay attention, on purpose, to the present moment. As described earlier, this is *mindfulness*. Often, we are caught in our thoughts about the past or predictions about the future, and we miss being in the here and now. I bet you know what this is like. Sometimes it feels like "zoning out," and, at other times, this mental distraction can feel emotionally charged. For example, if you're worried about an upcoming stressful event such as paying a bill, giving a presentation, or having a difficult conversation, the situation can feel all-consuming.

The antidote to this distraction is to practice bringing your attention back to the present moment over and over again, which is what you're going to do in this exercise. The benefit of this activity is that you are more likely to notice the sweet parts of life—the flower that you usually overlook on your evening walk, or the smell of coffee percolating in the morning—as well as things that need your attention, like the tenderness on your friend's face that signals she might need some care. This kind of practice—being present with what's happening right now—helps us savor life and respond more effectively when needed.

Debbie

You know that feeling you get when someone points out something "obvious" that you'd never noticed before in a familiar place? Maybe along a routine drive or walk, or inside a favorite store? Have you ever asked a grocery clerk where an item was only to find that you were standing right in front of it or had already passed it several times? Or have you walked into a room or opened a new web browser and totally forgotten why? I've certainly done these things, and I'm imagining you nodding and relating right about now. We all have those moments when we realize that our mind has been off somewhere else entirely because we were distracted.

All this might seem harmless, but if it happens frequently, it can affect how you perceive the world around you and how you feel emotionally. Getting lost in thought, whether you're ruminating about the past or worrying about the future, takes you out of the moment, causing you to miss out on so much of your life. You may overlook details about your experience, such as your child's laugh, your partner's loving glance, or a beautiful sunset. There were many times when I missed out on the full joy of a moment or didn't pick up on important details of an interaction with someone who really mattered to me.

There is a more skillful alternative. Once you start to notice the details of your experiences as they arise in the moment, you have the potential to boost your mood, be less forgetful, and miss out on fewer precious life events. This exercise will help you practice presence so that you are more fully living your life instead of just thinking about it.

Pick a time to take a short walk of about ten minutes. You can walk around your neighborhood, a local mall, the beach, a museum, or wherever you'd like.

Pretend that your Wise Woman is leading the way. What does she notice? What does she see, smell, taste, hear, feel?

Does your Wise Woman experience this walk any differently than you usually do? Did anything surprise you?

Take a few moments to journal your reflections on this experience with your Wise Woman.

_____

_____

_____

_____

_____

_____

_____

_____

_____

_____

_____

_____

List some upcoming opportunities for practicing mindful presence, such as:

- cooking

- completing a task at work

- having a conversation with a friend

_____

_____

_____

_____

_____

Write about how bringing mindful presence to these activities might improve your experiences and enrich your life in such moments.

_____

_____

_____

_____

_____

_____

_____

_____

Part 4

Connecting, Loving, and Boundaries

Having healthy, supportive relationships is vital to increased emotional and spiritual health. A sense of belonging to a community is fundamental to our well-being, yet this can be a challenging area for people who are emotionally sensitive or who have BPD traits. On a physical level, humans are highly interdependent and wouldn't survive without a large network of people working together to be sure we have food, shelter, and clothing. We are highly emotionally interdependent as well.

A sense of community reminds our nervous systems that we don't have to do it alone, that we have support, help, and, hopefully, a place to celebrate the gifts of life and grieve the losses. Belonging to a group helps us feel cared for and valued when life is good and when life is hard. Having the skills to maintain a sense of one's individual self, working through hard times in relationships, and being able to see another's perspective are all critical as community members.

For emotionally sensitive people, challenges around community and relationships can arise from having difficulty tolerating disagreement, not knowing how to repair a relationship after a rupture, or not knowing what, exactly, our needs are in a relationship or a group. You might find yourself feeling confused about what your role is in each of your relationships, which leads to unclear boundaries. You may not know how to balance differing needs between you and someone else, or how to establish a flow of give-and-take that works for you and the other person. You might have difficulty identifying what you need from a particular relationship. Left unaddressed, these challenges can lead to misunderstandings and disagreements that are damaging and do not accomplish the relationship repair and growth you want.

Being emotionally sensitive also means that you probably have strong *empathy* skills, which means that you have the capacity to be emotionally moved by another person's experiences and have a strong desire for connection with others. Empathy is the ability to not only relate to another person's experience but to actually *feel* their experience. People who are empathic and emotionally sensitive have the ability to deeply connect with another person's emotional tone, and this ability needs to be honed to be effective instead of dysregulating.

By tuning in to your Wise Woman, you can recenter back into your own experience instead of someone else's. With time and practice, your Wise Woman will be able to help you clarify whether what you are feeling are your emotions or your *mirror neurons* picking up signals from another person. Our nervous systems are wired to "mirror" other people, hence the name "mirror neurons" for the receptors throughout our bodies that gather information from our environment.

This ability to discern your own experiences, needs, and desire for closeness or distance is important in taking care of yourself and in preserving the health of your relationships. Practicing accessing your Wise Woman is essential in this domain because she has the ability to distinguish when a limit needs to be set, when to walk away from a situation or to confront it, and how to "cool down" before addressing hurt feelings.

In DBT, this is the process of moving from the emotional mind to our inner wisdom. When we are in an emotional state, usually we are activated and ready to react instead of mindfully respond. By practicing tuning in to our inner wisdom and felt physical sensations, we are better able to shift from an aroused, emotional feeling to a state of regulation, deeper breaths, and wider and wiser perspectives. Most relationship difficulties happen when we are in overly emotional or overly rational states. The key is to find a middle ground, a balance between honoring our emotions and looking at relationship issues with as much objectivity as possible as we consider multiple points of view.

Part 4 of this journal will help you get into the habit of listening to your Wise Woman to practice finding the balance of honoring your emotions, validating rational perspectives, and tuning in to a deeper level of intuitive awareness. Benefits may include noticing that your relationships feel supportive rather than chaotic, and nourishing rather than draining. The journal prompts in this section are designed to help you assess your relationships, explore your boundaries, and look at how to repair an important relationship after a rupture.

Relationship Inventory

Goal:

* ✸ Identify and evaluate current relationships

Kathryn

Relationships form the basis for emotional growth and healing. They can also wreak havoc on our lives if they are unsupportive or destructive. Taking an inventory of your relationships is a good first step in exploring what your support system looks like, who is in your life, and whether it's time to expand your circle of relationships.

Sometimes you might hold on to relationships that are toxic and draining simply because they are familiar. At other times you might not be aware of how many people you have in your life who are caring and enjoyable. This exercise is an opportunity to connect with your Wise Woman to help you take an honest look at whom you surround yourself with and why.

You'll be asked to look at your own patterns in relationships and to explore how they might need to change in order to get and maintain the relationships you need and desire. As Debbie describes in her story below, it's important to be gentle and nonjudgmental in this process, since relationships can bring up a host of thoughts and feelings.

Debbie

Years ago, I was sitting in a DBT group dreading the assignment we'd just been given. We were asked to list the important relationships in our lives by name and relationship type. For example, Keanu, boyfriend. Amber, friend. Elizabeth, therapist. I could feel a cold surge of adrenalin coursing through my veins. I was afraid of being humiliated when I was called upon to share my list because I had only three people on it. I imagined that all the other group members had long lists of friends and close family members that they could count on, and that I would look like a total loser because I didn't.

I was surprised as group members shared, because their lists were small too. A few things became clear from this experience. Because we were emotionally sensitive, easily dysregulated, and hadn't learned interpersonal skills, we had trouble creating and maintaining close bonds with others. Our DBT therapist wasn't trying to humiliate us with this assignment. She was illuminating that we all struggled similarly with relationships. We shared a deep desire to have meaningful, lasting connections with others in our lives, and we needed skills to help us bridge the gap between where we were and where we wanted to be. While drafting this list was a challenging exercise, acknowledging the support system I had made me feel grateful and inspired to grow it.

As you begin working on your list, I understand any apprehension you may be feeling. Know that I am extending my hand to hold yours as you do this important work.

Find a soothing place where you can focus. Start by taking a couple of deep breaths and tuning in to your Wise Woman as you begin writing.

List each of the important relationships in your life, noting the person's name and the relationship type (for example, "Will, brother").

_____

_____

_____

_____

_____

_____

_____

_____

Then, for each person on your list, answer the following:

What are the strengths of this relationship? What makes it work?

Is there a healthy reciprocity of giving and taking, listening and talking?

What are the weaknesses in this relationship?

What are some of the other person's and my behaviors that may threaten this relationship (for example, not being honest, backing out of commitments, angry outbursts, insecurity, frequent crises)?

Are there respectful boundaries?

Do I enjoy spending time with this person? If so, what do we do together?

How do I feel before and after spending time with this person?

Why is this relationship important to me? What does it add to my life?

_____

_____

_____

_____

_____

_____

_____

_____

_____

_____

_____

_____

_____

_____

_____

When you feel complete with your list, you might notice some patterns or have insights into your support system. Take some time to journal your reflections when you are done with your relationship inventory.

_____

_____

_____

_____

_____

_____

_____

_____

_____

_____

_____

_____

_____

_____

_____

_____

Beloved Boundaries
The Wisdom of Saying No

Goals:

* Identify the purpose of boundaries
* Identify where they are needed in relationships
* Explore how to set them

Kathryn

There's a saying about boundaries: "Good fences make good neighbors." The wisdom here is that people get along better when their personal spaces are clearly defined. When individuals are clear about their needs, limits, and feelings in a relationship, the relationship is healthier and easier to navigate. While it's not the focus of this workbook, it is important to remember that people with different amounts of sociocultural privilege—such as race, gender, sexuality, and background—experience different levels of permission to assert their boundaries.

So, what are *boundaries*, exactly? Boundaries are personal guidelines or limits that create safety in a relationship. When someone crosses your boundary, you might feel taken advantage of or violated. When you cross another person's boundary, he or she might have a similar reaction; the other person might even feel the need to push back or even end the relationship. This is one reason why knowing your own boundaries and limits is important as an emotionally sensitive person—they help create a safe zone for you and the other person.

The challenge with boundaries can be not knowing what your limits are, or not feeling able to establish them effectively. This exercise is focused on helping you become clearer about your boundaries and specifically about how to say *no* when a limit is being crossed. This can look like being asked to do something you don't have the time or energy to do, or continuing a relationship that isn't serving you anymore. This no is the boundary that comes from your Wise Woman. She might be saying, "No, my feelings *do* matter." Or "No, I don't want to pretend everything is fine when I feel taken advantage of."

As you do this work, keep in mind three common patterns that may be getting in the way of creating and setting boundaries:

1. **Worrying that you're being "mean" by setting boundaries or saying no to someone,** which causes you to avoid doing so altogether—and then you become passive in the relationship.

2. **Avoiding communicating your needs,** which can lead to becoming resentful of the other person. Resentment can unintentionally destroy a relationship.

3. **Not respecting the other person's boundaries,** which can lead to him or her needing to take a break from or ending the relationship.

Your Wise Woman is the part of you that is adept at knowing your boundaries, so tune in to your inner wisdom as you do this exercise. This practice will guide you in sensing your internal boundaries so that you are more effective at taking care of yourself in all of your relationships.

Debbie

If the thought of saying no to someone makes you feel super anxious, don't worry, you're not alone. I used to desperately avoid saying it. Even when I didn't want to, I said yes to all sorts of things, such as requests for my time (babysitting, covering someone's shift at work, cooking), even when I was tired or already overwhelmed with my own to-do list. I was afraid that if I said no to someone, he or she might reject me. It was an excruciatingly painful way to live. I didn't trust that I had the right to set a limit and refuse to do something if I didn't feel comfortable, didn't have time, or if I simply didn't want to do it. This all took a toll on my ability to regulate my emotions. My resentment would build toward those I wouldn't say no to, and then I'd eventually blow up at them. But as I got deeper into learning DBT and began setting and enforcing boundaries, my relationships became healthier. I gained confidence in my ability to convey my needs.

I'm happy to tell you that, most of the time, the dreaded fear that someone will stop liking you or even reject or leave you is unfounded. Sometimes you might notice a bit of surprise on the face of the person you say no to if the word is new in the relationship. But you might also find that the boundary is honored. You might find an increased feeling of esteem and self-respect that comes with honoring your limits and the other person doing the same. It doesn't always go this smoothly, though. There have been some relationships in my life that changed and some that ended when I became more assertive by setting boundaries and saying no.

This was initially heartbreaking, but it allowed me to see the relationships for what they were: if they were so fragile that my clear boundaries would be enough for the other person to leave, these weren't healthy, loving relationships to begin with. It can be a tough pill to swallow, but as you are getting more skillful and building the authentic life you want to live, you may find that dealing with the pain of ending such relationships sooner rather than later is in your best interest in the long run.

Exercise

It's time to think about your experience with boundaries. When you're ready, call upon your Wise Woman as you begin to journal through the following questions:

How do you define "boundaries," and what do they mean to you?

What are you unwilling to tolerate in a relationship? (This is your *no*, or limit, in terms of what you are willing to accept from another person and his or her behavior.)

When was the last time you set a boundary or said no in a relationship? If you haven't done this lately, is there a reason why?

How do you feel when saying no or setting a boundary? (If you cannot recall ever doing this, imagine what it might feel like.)

How do you feel when others set boundaries or express their limits? Is it painful, or do you appreciate them being clear about their needs?

In what situations and relationships do you have the hardest time asserting your boundaries or saying no (for example, with your significant other, your boss, your children, your parents)?

Are there situations or relationships that could benefit by you setting some boundaries? Will expressing your needs add anything to the relationship? Will this hurt the relationship?

"Visualize Your Boundaries." For a guided visualization on the state of your boundaries, visit http://www.newharbinger.com/40613.

As you consider these questions, you may discover actions you need to take, whether it's communicating your limits or repairing a relationship. If this is the case, take some time to journal from the perspective of your Wise Woman to figure out how to skillfully plan your next steps.

_____

_____

_____

_____

_____

_____

_____

_____

_____

_____

_____

_____

_____

_____

_____

_____

_____

Accepting a Different Point of View

Goal:

* Handle disagreements with less emotional suffering

Kathryn

Being able to tolerate and accept a difference of opinion is vital to maintaining any relationship. Yet for people who are emotionally sensitive, being able to stick with a relationship in the face of a disagreement or hurt feelings can be tricky. Often a disagreement can trigger you to move out of your balanced, centered Wise Woman and into an emotional state of mind. In this state, your emotions are running the show, and your ability to listen to the other person while also being gentle with yourself and your hurt feelings can be impaired.

This exercise is designed to help you notice when you shift from your Wise Woman—who knows how to navigate conflict more effectively—to an emotional state of mind, which reacts instead of skillfully responding to a situation. Knowing your patterns in relationships can help you practice being more alert to when you might need to pause and reconnect with your Wise Woman. It's also helpful to identify your habits so that you can practice new behaviors in the moment, which might mean taking deeper breaths before speaking or using some soothing self-talk before trying to resolve a dispute.

Debbie

Disagreements can trigger uncomfortable emotions and thoughts, and handling these can be very challenging, especially for people who are emotionally sensitive. Before learning DBT, it was hard for me to stay calm and in control when someone disagreed with me or pointed out something I could be doing better. I'd get very anxious and worried that, because we'd had a difference of opinion, no matter how small, he or she would reject or leave me because I was being difficult or because I wasn't perfect. The thought of being this vulnerable was terrifying, so I'd either disown my own perspective and adopt the other person's to avoid conflict, or I'd shut down, stop listening, and become defensive and sometimes even combative.

Reacting in these ways, of course, was counterproductive to my deep desire to build and keep healthy, lasting relationships. The good news is that there's a skillful way of handling these types of situations that transformed my relationships, and it's available to you too.

Instead of reacting in the moment by saying or doing something that may damage a relationship, you can choose to take time out and step away from an upsetting situation; then, you can come back to the interaction when you're feeling less fired up. When you return, keep in mind both the importance of hearing the other person, without interrupting, as well as the positive impact that expressing your perspective in a calm, gentle, and respectful manner can have on that person. This approach can go a long way toward creating and keeping the important relationships in your life. So let's practice by reflecting on a conversation that didn't go so well and gleaning some insights from your Wise Woman.

Exercise

Bring to mind a recent difference of opinion that caused you emotional distress. This experience may have been at work, school, home, or anywhere else. Describe this interaction in a couple sentences:

Now, tuning in to your Wise Woman, use the following prompts to guide your journaling:

What did you feel physically, emotionally, and energetically in this interaction?

What was going on that led up to this interaction? (This might be something that happened earlier in the day that made you more vulnerable to becoming distressed.)

In this interaction, what did you want to do? In other words, what was your impulse? Did you notice an urge to interrupt, become defensive, or to stop listening? An impulse to retreat or avoid or freeze?

What were the thoughts, worries, or concerns that you noticed during the discussion?

If this interaction didn't go well, how could it have gone better?

How can you be more mindfully present in your next disagreement (for example, taking a pause before speaking, breathing, allowing the other person to complete his or her thoughts without interrupting, being respectful and kind while sharing your own perspective, suggesting working together to come to a compromise that works for both of you)?

_____

_____

_____

_____

_____

_____

_____

_____

_____

_____

_____

_____

_____

_____

_____

_____

Repairing Relationships
Mending After a Rupture

Goals:

- ✳ Explore the potential for repairing a damaged relationship
- ✳ Assess whether you want to take steps to repair
- ✳ Explore how to communicate after a rupture in a relationship

Kathryn

The idea of repairing a relationship is completely foreign to some people. I often hear this from clients when we are assessing whether a rupture is final or not. That you could make a relationship better than it was before someone was hurt, offended, or criticized is a concept many people were never taught. A repair in a relationship after a falling-out is more than an apology—it is an apology with action *and* intention. A repair comes from your Wise Woman with the intention of making the relationship even stronger.

We all know the difference between someone saying sorry out of a sense of obligation and saying it with heartfelt intent, which is when someone has actually taken the time to consider how the other person felt in an interaction and how to prevent repeating the offense in the future. The impact is so much greater when someone means it and is willing to make a change for the health of the relationship.

If you have been hurt or have hurt someone, it can take time to consider whether a repair is in order. It makes sense to think about your values in the relationship, if the relationship is worth it to you to take the time and energy necessary to rectify it, and if you even want to do so. A repair means opening your heart, and that can be challenging and vulnerable, regardless of whether you are on the giving or receiving end.

This exercise guides you in considering the pros and cons of mending a relationship. You will consult with your Wise Woman about how to initiate a repair.

Debbie

During the many years that I struggled to manage my emotions, I behaved in ways that damaged and destroyed very important relationships in my life. Not only did I not know how to handle the intense emotions that sometimes came up in relationships, I also didn't know how to go about repairing those relationships once damage had been done. I didn't know healthy ways to express my remorse and ask for another chance. Instead, I'd panic, feel desperate, and end up pushing the person farther away by relentlessly calling, texting, emailing, and begging for forgiveness.

I had an experience like this with an ex-boyfriend many moons ago. It was very difficult for me to accept the painful reality that the man I loved no longer wanted to be with me. At first, I pleaded with him to reconsider, but when that didn't work, I began to act desperately. I sent lots of emails. Lots of texts. Lots of voicemails.

Thinking back, my behavior reminds me of a meme showing a woman talking on the phone with the caption "I'm just going to send you a thousand messages to prove to you how normal I am." I was panicking, and I didn't have the skills to cope with the emotions I was feeling or to behave appropriately with the other person by honoring his boundaries. Instead of convincing him to give me another chance, I pushed him farther and farther away.

Eventually I stopped messaging him. I focused on other things and surrounded myself with friends and family and activities. Months later, without the charge of the intense emotions, my ex-boyfriend came to mind. I decided to call him to let him know I was genuinely sorry and ask for his forgiveness. He granted it. I didn't get everything I wanted (getting back together with him), but because I was truly ready to express my remorse, take responsibility for my behaviors that led to the breakup and my boundary-pushing behavior afterward, I received his acceptance of my apology.

I was fortunate that things turned out well. Sometimes they don't. Sometimes the other person will not be ready or willing to accept your apology or make amends. There is a possibility that, even if you genuinely express remorse and offer to do what you can to repair any damage that was done, the other person may not be receptive. This can be very painful, and, in this case, you'll need to call upon some of your other skills (particularly around tolerating distress and using self-care) to manage the emotions that may arise. No matter what happens, I think you're very brave for being willing to put yourself out there and being vulnerable by saying you are sorry.

Before you approach the other person with your apology, make sure you're ready. It may be too soon for you to say you're sorry if you:

- are feeling anxious and are tempted to try to just patch things over quickly,

- haven't fully thought through your role and responsibility in the rupture, or

- aren't ready to present a heartfelt apology and your intention to not repeat the offense.

Note: In twelve-step-program literature, there is a step focused on making amends. The caution is to only attempt to do so when it will not cause more harm than good to the other person. The short and plain of it: if you think making amends will hurt anyone, don't do it; instead, consider how you can come to internal peace with your own behavior.

Exercise

Begin by settling into a calm, quiet space and taking a few deep breaths to connect to your Wise Woman. You might even put one hand on your stomach or heart and close your eyes briefly before you start writing.

Journal your answers to the questions below to help you slow down and decide when and how to proceed. From the voice of your Wise Woman, answer the following questions:

Is there a relationship in your life that is in need of a repair?

What has happened to make you feel as though a repair is needed? Was there a disagreement? Disappointment? Hurt feelings? What information tells you a repair is needed?

Are you the one who needs to initiate the repair? (Did you contribute to the rupture?) What was your role in this situation? Do you feel ready to take responsibility or do you need time, support, or communication? Notice what would be supportive as you consider this step of initiation if you were in the wrong.

Do you need the other person to join in mending the relationship, especially if he or she was the cause of the problem? What would you like to hear from him or her? Is there anything the other person needs to do to demonstrate the repair beyond words?

What are the pros and cons of repairing the relationship?

Is the relationship worth repairing?

Are your values in alignment with this relationship?

Are your needs being met in the relationship?

How do you feel before and after interacting with the other person?

If you decide that a repair is in order, what does your Wise Woman need in order to follow through?

How might she communicate this to the other person? Consider tone of voice, body language, as well as word choice.

Do you think the other person will be receptive? If not, how do you plan to take care of yourself and stay skillful during and after the interaction?

What do you need to do to make amends?

Take your time with the last question—you might consider writing out an imaginary back-and-forth dialogue between your Wise Woman and the other person to explore this exercise even deeper.

_____

_____

_____

_____

_____

Part 5

Setting Intentions and Ideas for Future Exploration

As an emotionally sensitive person, you might find it challenging to see your future in a hopeful light. When you have a history of inner and outer turmoil, it's understandable that you'd be skeptical. Hopefully, you're already seeing that it *is* possible to shift from existing in chaos to living a life that feels balanced, fulfilled, and stable. You may have arrived at the beginning of this journaling process in that place of chaos. Because of the inner work you've completed in these pages, your belief in your ability to continue to grow and heal is now likely increasing, allowing you to move away from skepticism and ever closer toward the life you want to live.

We trust that the time you've spent with this journal has helped you unearth many helpful insights about your emotions, thoughts, goals, and relationships. We congratulate you for your willingness to dive so deep into your experience with such honesty and bravery! As these pages and our time together wrap up, it's time to set your intentions for continuing your healing journey beyond this book.

In part 5, you'll foster continued connection with your Wise Woman to build the future you want and to develop even more emotional resiliency. Your Wise Woman can see beyond your fears of repeating the past and can present a clearer picture of your desired—and attainable—future. She lives deeper than the fight-flight-freeze response of the brain and can guide you in setting and keeping intentions and goals for the short and long term.

Remember this truth: *People with emotional sensitivity have a superpower. Once their emotional energy is skillfully channeled, they are highly intuitive, creative, and able to create lives of beauty and power.*

The final part of this book is designed to remind you of your superpower so that you can move forward in your life with strength and continued insight.

Using Imagination to Access Inner Wisdom

Goals:

* Strengthen confidence in your inner wisdom

* Practice accessing inner wisdom through visualization

* Begin strengthening neural pathways of resilient coping through visualization

Kathryn

We already know that the brain is highly malleable and can rewire and repair itself with focused intention and practice. But did you know that this healing is possible through something as simple as using your imagination? *Active imagination* is a visualization technique that creates and strengthens new neural pathways in the brain while utilizing the power of your imagination. You can use it as a tool to access your Wise Woman, as she is often overlooked by habitual thinking patterns. It can also be used to gather insight into your life. Active imagination is not the same thing as passive daydreaming or zoning out. This practice, while creative, is focused and intentional.

Sometimes when people are just beginning DBT and we discuss listening to their own Wise Woman—rather than strictly to their emotions or thoughts—they look at me slightly dumbfounded. I often hear self-doubt and self-criticism about how they must not have access to the same wisdom as other people or that something is simply "wrong" with them. However, when I guide people through this experience, they often come out of it surprised at how clear and simple it is to begin listening to their Wise Woman and how quickly this skill can be mastered.

Throughout this book you've begun to envision and connect with your Wise Woman. The following practice will lead you through an active imagination where you will encounter your *future self*—your Wise Woman within who has traveled farther down the DBT path and gained many valuable insights along the way. You will have the chance to practice consulting her guidance, wisdom, and insight. Whatever happens, remember that you have access to this wisdom whenever you need it, and you can give this exercise a try as often as you desire.

Treat this practice as an experimental journey into your own imagination. You cannot do this wrong. Let this practice be playful instead of serious, to help your brain and nervous system relax. When you feel calm and relatively safe, you are in the best condition for your brain to try something new. Journaling about your experience is an effective way to reinforce and anchor your imaginative practice, so use the prompts to guide you as you write.

Debbie

I absolutely love this type of activity for one main reason. I used to really struggle with *catastrophizing*. When something upsetting would happen, my mind would often race toward worrying that the worst possible scenario in the history of mankind was surely on its way. Of course, this led to a lot of anxiety and suffering, and most of the time the outcomes I dreaded never happened! One day I realized that the same imagination that can scare me out of my wits can also be channeled in positive, constructive, and healthier ways.

Active imagination allows you to experience a cool blend of art (your imagination is limitless in its ability to create) and science (as Kathryn mentioned, you are truly rewiring your brain and calming your nervous system with this work). You might notice that you feel incredibly relaxed and soothed afterward—two great motivating factors that'll keep you coming back to this exercise often.

I encourage you to tap into your creative mind. Allow yourself to vividly envision the imagery in the prompts below, and take your time with it. I highly recommend that you find a quiet space where you will not be disturbed. Dim the lights, turn off your devices, and allow yourself to become fully immersed in this activity. Enjoy!

Exercise

"Using Imagination to Access Inner Wisdom." To hear a guided version of this exercise, visit http://www.newharbinger.com/40613. Begin by thinking of a place that you find nourishing or relaxing. Take several moments to allow your body and mind to slow down and come to a sense of calm while holding this place in mind. When you feel more at ease and are taking deeper breaths, you are ready to begin your visualization.

You can keep your eyes open and relaxed or closed. You can also journal through the visualization as it comes to you if that will help you stay focused.

Start by bringing to mind an image of your future self. Imagine that she is wise, resilient, and has cultivated some amazing strengths throughout her life.

Notice what she looks like. How old is she? What is she wearing? Does she look familiar? Take a second to simply notice this image in front of you.

Next, imagine that you start to speak to her. What do you want to ask? Does she have something to tell you? If there is something you've been struggling with, see if you can ask for guidance and notice her response.

Allow this interaction to go on for as long as you desire until it naturally comes to a close. Say good-bye and give thanks for anything you received from your future self.

When your practice is complete, take several minutes to write down your experience, thoughts, and insights that arose. You could even draw a picture of what you saw and experienced.

_____

_____

_____

_____

_____

_____

_____

_____

_____

_____

_____

_____

_____

Assessing Your Values

Goals:

* Evaluate how you spend your time, energy, money, and attention

* Assess if your behavior is in line with what you most value

* Explore any changes that would help bring your behavior in alignment with your values

Kathryn

Identifying your *values*, your own personal code of conduct, can help skillfully guide your behavior and decision-making when life feels confusing or chaotic. While culture, society, and family often implicitly define which ideals should be most important to us (for example, focusing on family first, or being a hard worker, or being honest above all else), we as individuals also develop our own personal set of virtues and values that we live by based on who we are, what we enjoy, and what brings purpose to our lives. Your values function as an inner road map that guides you toward which way to go and which choices to make as you navigate the world to build a satisfying life.

When you live your life in alignment with the principles you most value, anxiety and stress decrease. Why? Because you experience less of a disconnect between who you want to be and the choices you make from moment to moment. (For example, if you identify being honest and loyal as important values, and you go about your day refraining from telling little white lies, by day's end you'll likely be happier with yourself and in your relationships than if you'd gone against your values and told lies.) This doesn't mean life is necessarily any easier or less filled with challenges, but it does mean that you are more connected to your inner compass. When you live in accordance with your values, your decisions stem from you consulting your personal code of conduct, not from your emotionally charged, impulsive reactions.

Often when I work with clients who are in the midst of a big life decision or who are plagued with chronic ambivalence, we take plenty of time to assess which choices or actions they could take that are most in alignment with who they want to be in the world. This helps them approach the problem from their Wise Woman, and usually the decision arises spontaneously and with much less effort than trying to force an outcome through purely rational means.

The following practice is designed to help bring awareness to the values that matter most to you, not just what you think should be important to you. There is no judgment about what your values are, and the purpose of this exercise is to increase your awareness about why you do what you do so that you can consciously build a life that is meaningful. In DBT, a main goal is to help you create the life you want to live rather than the one you'd rather avoid or escape. Discovering what you value and referring to it often is a powerful tool in this journey of leading a life that feels satisfying to you, not someone else.

Debbie

I absolutely love this approach to discovering what you value without judgment. In a class with my spiritual coach recently, we were asked to write down what we do with our leisure time. I noted that I spend a lot of time watching television in the evening. It's not something I didn't know, but my initial reaction seeing it on paper was self-judgment and criticism: *I guess I value being a lazy, zoned-out sloth.* Then I did what this exercise invites you to do. I looked at how I spend my time in the evening from a place of nonjudgment and curiosity. This really shifted how I felt about it and gave me valuable insight into how this behavior ties into my values.

I am a creative, giving person, and I work hard and expend a lot of mental energy during the day. In the evening, depending on how intense and busy my day was, I enjoy watching anything, from a lighthearted black-and-white TV show to an intense drama or sci-fi series. My time in the evening watching TV involves me being in my pajamas, reclined cozily on the couch in a blanket cocoon with my cats and usually some dark chocolate. It's a time of self-nurturing and rest.

I value self-care and rest, and doing the values exercise helped me get in touch with this and consider other ways I can honor this value if I want to mix it up and not watch television on a given night (like going for a pedicure or a massage or a meal out).

Approach this exercise openly. No judgments. No wrong answers. Just reflect and use any information you gather to help you live a life that feels good and in alignment with your values.

Exercise

Begin by finding a place of calm in your body and mind. Make an inner agreement that you will practice curiosity instead of self-judgment as you assess your values.

Make a list of all the people, places, things, events, and experiences that you enjoy, that make you feel nourished, or that you simply love. This list can be long or short. Simply take your time to notice what in your life brings you joy.

_____

_____

_____

_____

_____

_____

_____

_____

_____

_____

_____

_____

_____

_____

_____

_____

_____

_____

_____

_____

Next, make a list of the top five places you spend your money. This is not where your money *should* go, it's where it actually goes.

_____

_____

_____

_____

_____

Then, make a list of the top five places you spend your time. Again, this is not where you *should* spend your time, it's what you actually do.

_____

_____

_____

_____

_____

Make a list of the top five things you think about. What is consistently running through your mind?

_____

_____

_____

_____

_____

When you have these four lists complete, take a look and notice if you see any patterns emerging. Tune in to your Wise Woman and ask if she can highlight the values that will shape your personal code of conduct for living in integrity based on what you enjoy, how you behave, and what you think about. What did you notice about these lists? Did anything stand out to you? Were you surprised by any similarities or differences between your lists of how you spend your time, money, and thinking? Based on these lists, what does it look like you value most? Is this different than what you feel to be true to your Wise Woman? Write down what you discover about your values, what they mean to you, and why.

What's at Stake?

Goals:

* Identify how you can benefit from your ongoing introspection, skills practice, and journaling

* Link your goals to your deeper values and desires

* Explore your motivations

Kathryn

We can have all the facts, reasons for change, and mental motivation for why to sustain change, but if these motivations are based exclusively in our rational experience and are disconnected from our deeper needs and desires, change is not going to maintain itself. We know from research that if motivation is not in some way tied to our deeper values, we will go back to old patterns and behaviors (Cameron 2014). It's not enough to think our way to change. We need to feel it. This is where all of your practice with accessing your Wise Woman comes in.

It's also true that while you can practice as many DBT skills as you want and do them "perfectly," if you don't have a deeper sense of why you're practicing these skills, you might end up going through the motions of your life instead of growing, enjoying, and savoring your life (Cameron 2014). This is an important and interesting step in DBT: moving into a life worth living. The difference is that your life is connected to a sense of purpose, intention, and pleasure, which is part of the healing and growth process. We are now exploring your motivation for change from a place of wisdom rather than desperation.

In this practice you are going to explore your motivation from the perspective of your Wise Woman. What is most important to her in terms of sustaining change and engaging in new behaviors? What does your Wise Woman most want you to know as you explore moving forward with new practices and patterns? In this exercise, allow yourself to imagine what is necessary for your life to flourish and for you to feel alive and satisfied, along with the behaviors needed to get you there.

Debbie

There will be moments along your healing path when you'll be presented with opportunities that look really good on paper (and resonate with your reasonable, rational mind), yet you'll experience some hesitation from your heart (your inner wisdom). It's important to listen to both sides of your experience when this happens, because, as Kathryn says, it takes more than rational logic to build a life worth living.

A few years ago, while teaching at DBT Path, I was also working a full-time job. It paid well, and I received lots of validation for my work. But these benefits were not enough to sustain my motivation beyond about a year of being in that position. My values were becoming more and more apparent to me. I wanted to be of service in a different way, and I knew that I would need to make some changes to make that happen and to truly be living a life worth living.

I tapped into my inner wisdom and used DBT skills to sort out how to make that happen. I sketched out the pros and cons of leaving the job to focus on teaching others skills. In the end, I decided to take the risk, and I am happy that I did. It was scary at first, but I knew that I was feeling unsettled and discontented by only listening to my logical brain's preference that I receive a steady salary and stay an employee. I had to listen to my heart as well. I did so with caution and with lots of consulting with mentors, and then I made the leap. This is an example of how listening to my deeper motivations and values shaped my behavior and choices, leading to greater and sustaining fulfillment. This is when DBT helps shift us from simply using the skills to get through life to actually *building* the lives we want to live.

Exercise

Begin this practice by centering yourself in your body and the present moment. You may mentally or verbally invite your Wise Woman to show up as you begin your journaling practice.

Start by making a list of the people in your life who matter to you. These are the people you love and care about, and who love and care about you in return. You can also include pets on this list.

_____

_____

_____

_____

_____

_____

_____

_____

_____

Next to each name, write why it matters to your relationship that you continue your journey of healing and recovery.

Next, make a list of your long- and short-term goals in the following domains of your life:

Relationships: What do you desire for your relationships in the short term? How about long term?

_____

_____

_____

_____

_____

_____

_____

Education: Do you have any desires or goals for expanding your knowledge? What might that look and feel like?

_____

_____

_____

_____

_____

_____

Career: What are your short- and long-term goals for your work and career? Does your Wise Woman have any insight into bringing your gifts more fully into the world?

_____

_____

_____

_____

_____

_____

_____

Housing: Are you satisfied with your home and housing situation? If so, how might you make it even more satisfying? If not, what needs to change?

_____

_____

_____

_____

_____

_____

_____

Emotional well-being and mental health: What is important for your life in terms of your inner experience and mental well-being? What do you need to do to maintain or increase your health?

_____

_____

_____

_____

_____

_____

_____

Physical health: How do you want to feel physically in the short and long term? What will help you feel that or get there?

_____

_____

_____

_____

_____

_____

_____

Refer to this list to remind yourself why the transformational work you're doing, though it's sometimes incredibly challenging, is ultimately totally worth it.

Building Mastery
Challenging Yourself
with Small Steps

Goal:

✹ Create a daily self-care routine to continue
implementing after you've completed this journal,
led by your Wise Woman

Kathryn

Remember how Rome wasn't built in a day? Well, building a life
worth living is the same idea. We don't simply wake up one morning
to see that our life has magically transformed. In fact, it's the small,
daily, and seemingly insignificant steps of challenging ourselves and
trying new things that make all the difference as we build lives that
we could hardly conceive of months before our hard work
commenced.

While we don't want to encourage the "no pain, no gain" men-
tality, it is necessary to push your *growth edges* to extend beyond your
life as it is now. Your growth edge is the place where you feel both
slightly uncomfortable *and* slightly excited about trying something
new. In DBT, when you allow yourself to confront and push past your
growth edges by trying new skills that might initially feel unfamiliar,
you allow yourself to build *mastery*. The concept of building mastery
is vital in DBT because it means that you feel competent, capable,
and confident in your ability to use skills and move past previous

unskillful ways of living your life. For example, a growth edge for me has been to practice using my voice and sharing my opinions even when I feel nervous or unsure of myself. Over time and with practice, I've become much more articulate and self-assured in having challenging conversations.

This practice is focused on helping you notice your unique growth edges and setting intentions to continue confronting areas of challenge. The goal is to build mastery in your life. Remember that learning and change are best accomplished when you aren't overly stressed. And be sure to celebrate every small victory—this will help you notice each step forward, no matter how tiny, and will prevent overwhelm by focusing on what is working instead of how far you have to go.

Debbie

As I've continued to grow and heal in my recovery from BPD, I've read a number of self-help books, taken personal development and spiritual growth courses, and worked with a life coach. Why? Because I want to continue to grow! As you're likely beginning to experience for yourself, learning and practicing DBT skills and befriending your Wise Woman opens you up to discovering who you are, the gifts you bring to this world, and insights on how to build a life that is worth living to *you*. This is exciting! It motivates you to discover ways to bring meaning to your life and to take active steps toward these things. Through being mindfully aware of your emotions, thoughts, and needs, you'll naturally begin to identify areas in your life where you can challenge yourself and stretch those growth edges.

Some challenging aspects of my life where I've stretched my growth edges had to do with activities I was very afraid to do in the past (but desperately wanted to do!): video calls, going to dance classes, and getting trained as a life coach, to name a few. Pushing past anxiety to participate in video calls has deepened the intimacy of conversations I have with people who aren't nearby; going to dance classes helps me with my goal of being more graceful and mindful in my body; and getting trained as a life coach allows me to serve my students and humanity (and myself!) in a deeper capacity than I could without the training. Now it's time for you to think about the aspects you want to stretch and grow. Have fun with this!

Exercise

Take a few moments to sit in a quiet space, close your eyes, and take in a few cleansing, slow-paced breaths. Ask your Wise Woman for guidance with noticing your growth edges and setting goals for yourself.

Begin by writing down your responses to the following prompts:

Ask your Wise Woman where you desire to grow in your life. Where can you sense a "growth edge" (that place where you feel both nervous *and* excited for change)? This could be setting boundaries in relationships, taking a step toward a long-held dream, or using a self-care skill every day.

Example: I can feel that I really want to be able to sustain relationships in my life. So even though it feels so strange to me now, my growth edge is to "check the facts" whenever I feel betrayed by a friend before I confront him or her.

_____

_____

_____

_____

_____

_____

_____

_____

_____

_____

_____

_____

_____

_____

_____

Consider your motivation to work toward your goal and to push through your growth edge. Why is this goal important to you? What would be different about your life if you succeeded?

Example: If I were able to delay reacting to feeling betrayed by my friends, then I would have more stable friendships. This would feel really good because I would have people to do things with on the weekends and people to call when I'm upset or need support.

_____

_____

_____

_____

_____

_____

_____

_____

_____

_____

_____

_____

_____

_____

What do you need to do today to start working toward your goal? Make this something small, measurable, and specific.

Example: Today I am going to review the section in this book on "checking the facts" and remind myself what that skill means.

_____

_____

_____

_____

_____

_____

_____

_____

_____

_____

_____

_____

_____

_____

_____

_____

What do you need to do each day to work toward your goal? If you hit roadblocks or obstacles, what is your plan to continue moving forward?

Example: I'm going to write my goal on a sticky note and put it on my bathroom mirror. I will look at my goal every day to remind myself to practice delaying acting on my emotions in relationships, especially if they are telling me to do something that would end the relationship. If I hit an obstacle, I will wait one day before deciding to give up, and I'll remind myself of all the ways I've succeeded over the past month to work toward my goal.

_____

_____

_____

_____

_____

_____

_____

_____

_____

_____

_____

_____

_____

Feel free to complete this practice with other goals as well. Here is a template you can use right now, or go to http://www.newharbin ger.com/40613 and download a PDF that you can use anytime.

My goal is: _____

_____

_____

_____

My motivation to achieve this goal is: _____

_____

_____

_____

One thing I will do every day to work toward this goal is: _____

_____

_____

_____

My plan for when I hit an obstacle is: _____

_____

_____

_____

_____

My goal is: _____

_____

_____

_____

My motivation to achieve this goal is: _____

_____

_____

_____

One thing I will do every day to work toward this goal is: _____

_____

_____

_____

My plan for when I hit an obstacle is: _____

_____

_____

_____

_____

My goal is: _____

_____

_____

_____

My motivation to achieve this goal is: _____

_____

_____

_____

_____

One thing I will do every day to work toward this goal is: _____

_____

_____

_____

My plan for when I hit an obstacle is: _____

_____

_____

_____

_____

Moving Forward
with Intention

Goals:

- ✳ Reflect on and plan for the future
- ✳ Set an intention for moving toward goals
- ✳ Set an intention to release old hurts and mistakes
- ✳ Access self-compassion and gentleness

Kathryn

About once every three months I have a practice of sitting down with my journal, lighting a candle, and taking time to assess my life. Often there's an area I'm sensing needs some attention, whether it's relationships, work, finances, or a bubbling desire for a fun weekend getaway. This practice of slowing down to reflect and reconnect with *why* I do what I do, and whether I need to readjust something according to my values, helps me maintain inner balance and feel good about my choices.

In the midst of keeping up with the busyness and emotional needs of day-to-day living, my clients often tell me that they've lost track of what brings them joy and what they want to contribute to the world beyond simply surviving. I encourage you to use this practice as a regular reflection opportunity to reconnect with your goals, what makes you feel alive, and the life you want to lead so that you're not just surviving but thriving.

Sometimes this practice of reflection and intention setting brings clarity that a particular relationship, a painful memory, or a story we keep retelling about ourselves needs to be released for us to move forward. While this is easier said than done, this exercise can help you clarify what, if anything, needs to be let go to welcome in the new.

You might also discover that you're generally on track in terms of living a life that feels meaningful and satisfying, but a little extra self-care or time to savor the small things is all that's needed. So whatever you find is needing your attention, release any judgments that may come up and choose to honor the wisdom of your writing.

In this practice, you will reconnect with your future self to receive a letter, from her to you, in this present moment. Consider this letter a gift and a message from a part of yourself that has coped well, succeeded in some way, or overcome a challenge. This will, hopefully, give you some insight about your life as it is now and what you can do to move toward your goals.

Debbie

This is such an empowering exercise, as it's a very gentle gateway into believing in and trusting your inner wisdom. Often, we seek counsel from someone else when we feel in need of guidance on a life issue. This exercise allows you to turn inward instead and generate your own self-guidance from your truest, highest self, and not from an outside source.

Over the years, I've used oracle cards to help me tap into my inner wisdom. I ask a question, draw a card, and then look at the imagery as I would a Rorschach test image. The Rorschach test uses ink blot patterns on paper, and the subject is asked to say what he or she sees in the image. A mental health professional then interprets the response. When I draw an oracle card and come up with my interpretation, I then empower *myself* and trust that *my* interpretation is a result of me accessing my Wise Woman.

Think of the exercise below as a tool to assist you in tapping into your inner wisdom. Each time you practice, your confidence in your ability to answer your own needs and take even better care of yourself will grow. And, setting up your space for the practice can feel particularly nurturing and soothing. You could, like me, even use oracle cards as you ask yourself the questions, if you feel so inclined. Enjoy!

Exercise

To begin this exercise, take a moment to create a space that feels intentional and cared for. This can be as simple as lighting a candle, choosing soothing music, or placing a meaningful object next to your journal. Then, take a couple of soothing breaths and reconnect with your future self. Bring her to mind as you did in the exercise titled "Using Imagination to Access Inner Wisdom."

When you feel connected to your future self, take some time to write a letter from her perspective to you, as you are in this moment. You can come up with your own letter or fill in the blanks of this template. You can also go to http://www.newharbinger.com/40613 and download a PDF that you can use anytime. Remember, you are writing from the perspective of your future Wise Woman.

Dear _____ [your name],

This is what I would like you to know about your life right

now: _____

_____

_____

_____.

I can see that you are struggling with _____

_____

_____

_____ [a stressor or problem

you are facing]. Here is my guidance for this situation:

_____

_____

_____

_____

_____

_____

_____

_____

_____

_____.

Something I suggest you consider releasing or letting go in order to move forward is _____

_____

_____

_____

_____.

What you can focus on more is _____

_____

_____ [maybe a daily practice or a long-term goal].

What is important for you to remember in building a meaningful, joyful life is _____

_____

_____.

Where you could use some self-compassion is _____

_____

_____

_____.

With love,

Your Future Self

_____

_____

_____

_____

_____

_____

_____

_____

_____

_____

_____

_____

_____

_____

_____

_____

Remember, there is no "right way" to do this exercise, and this letter might be very long or quite to the point. Practice being non-judgmental and staying open to hearing your inner wisdom. To complete this exercise, you might even mail this letter to yourself to receive a gift like no other!

Moving On and Moving Forward

Sometimes, upon reaching the end of a journey, perhaps like your encounter with this journal, you suddenly realize you have only just begun. We hope this is your experience and that this journal is simply the first phase of a long, nurturing, and exciting relationship you will continue to cultivate with your own Wise Woman, your inner wisdom. The essence of this work is to be able to trust yourself, to be able to tap into your power and insight whenever you desire without permission from anyone else.

The importance of discovering and following your own inner compass cannot be underestimated. When you feel a sense of permission to access and trust your own inner wisdom, this allows you to show up in the world in ways you cannot imagine. Some of the ways we, your guides through this journal, have experienced these changes is through healing of relationships, a deeper sense of purpose in the world, greater ability to take leaps toward our highest values, and creating lives that are meaningful and fulfilling. Before this journey of self-trust and self-care, life can feel bleak and uninspiring. While trusting your own inner wisdom doesn't cure the ails of the world, it certainly does open up a wealth of options that were previously unavailable or unrecognizable. We hope that you continue to utilize the skills, insights, and practices you explored in this journal.

Perhaps you have established a routine of daily or weekly journaling and are apprehensive about missing this sacred time with yourself. Don't stop. You can always come back to the exercises and re-explore them in a new, blank journal as many times as you'd like. You're likely to gain new insights and perspectives each time you do the exercises as you continue to grow and evolve. There will be days when you may also spontaneously just know what would be helpful to write, without any prompt. Trust this spontaneity—it is your Wise Woman guiding you in writing that is helpful, whether you need to process an emotional event, discover the best decision in a difficult situation, reflect upon your progress being skillful, or savor a triumphant experience.

Keep up the great work you've been doing. You are worth it. And we are honored to have been a part of your journey. Stay strong, Wise Woman.

Acknowledgments

From Debbie

I am so grateful to the amazing people (and animals!) in my life who showed me support and love while writing this workbook with Kathryn. Thanks to all of you, including but not limited to: my family; my dear friends and loved ones; my students; my book and blog readers; social media followers; PK, for all the deep work we're doing together; Charis Lynn; and, of course, Kathryn, my amazing collaborator on this project. Thank you to Spirit for reminding me who I really am and guiding me in my purpose on this planet in this incarnation.

From Kathryn

This book would not have happened if it were not for the wise, embodied, and powerful women in my life who taught me how to listen to my own inner wisdom. I'm deeply grateful for my friends, family, and council of mentors and ancestors supporting my work and this project. Thank you to Debbie for such a fun and satisfying collaboration, and to all of those who will find empowerment in these pages. I am also indebted to the brilliance and healing of my clients, whom I am privileged to walk alongside and who inspire me every day.

References

Aguirre, B. A., and G. Galen. 2013. *Mindfulness for Borderline Personality Disorder: Relieve Your Suffering Using the Core Skill of Dialectical Behavior Therapy.* Oakland, CA: New Harbinger Publications.

American Psychiatric Association. 2013. *Diagnostic and Statistical Manual of Mental Disorders*, 5th ed. Arlington, VA: American Psychiatric Publishing.

Cameron, A., K. Palm Reed, and B. Gaudiano. 2014. "Addressing Treatment Motivation in Borderline Personality Disorder: Rationale for Incorporating Values-Based Exercises into Dialectical Behavior Therapy." *Journal of Contemporary Psychotherapy* 44 (2): 109–116.

Deliens, G., M. Gilson, and P. Peigneux. 2014. "Sleep and the Processing of Emotions." *Experimental Brain Research* 232 (5): 1,403–1,414.

Linehan, Marsha M. 1993. *DBT® Skills Training Manual, Second Edition.* New York: The Guilford Press.

Maccari, L., D. Martella, A. Marotta, N. Sebastiani, N. Banaj, L. J. Fuentes, and M. Casagrande. 2014. "Effects of Sleep Loss on Emotion Recognition: A Dissociation Between Face and Word Stimuli." *Experimental Brain Research* 232 (10): 3,147–3,157.

Osowiecka, M. 2016. "An Artist Without Wings? Regulation of Emotions Through Aesthetic Experiences." *Creativity: Theories–Research–Applications* 3(1): 94–103.

Wineman, P. A. 2009. "The Efficacy of a Dialectical Behavior Therapy-Based Journal-Writing Group with Inpatient Adolescent Females: Improving Emotion Regulation, Depressive Symptoms and Suicidal Ideation." *Dissertation Abstracts International* 70: 3,817.

Debbie Corso is a mental health blogging pioneer, courageously chronicling her journey while lighting a torch to provide hope to a severely emotionally wounded community. She has a BS in behavioral science, communications, and English from the New York Institute of Technology in interdisciplinary studies, as well as a certificate in early childhood development. She is a certified Emotional Confidence Life Coach, and is also in recovery from borderline personality disorder (BPD).

Through hard, consistent work using dialectical behavior therapy (DBT), she no longer meets the criteria to be considered "borderline." Her work as an intake coordinator and case manager at a nonprofit organization, working closely with children at risk for abuse and neglect, was the catalyst that propelled her to document and share her powerful journey through her blog, and hopeful and encouraging books on overcoming the oppressive symptoms of BPD. She currently cofacilitates worldwide DBT psychoeducational courses online at www.emotionallysensitive.com, and is author of *Stronger Than BPD*. Corso resides in Northern California.

Kathryn C. Holt, MSSW, LCSW, is a psychotherapist who accompanies people on the journey of reclaiming their hunger, desire, and permission to live fully in their bodies and lives. She writes about her journey and her psychospiritual approach to healing at www.kathryncholt.com. Kathryn studied DBT at Columbia University in New York City, NY, and worked with teens, adults, and families using DBT prior to moving to Boulder, CO, where she now lives and practices. She is now pursuing her PhD in depth psychology, and offers individual therapy, groups, and retreats with the intention of reconnecting people with their power, wisdom, and purpose.

Foreword writer **Kiera Van Gelder, MFA**, is an artist, educator, and writer diagnosed with BPD. An international speaker and advocate, she is featured in the documentary *Back from the Edge: Living with and Recovering from Borderline Personality Disorder*.

MORE BOOKS *from*
NEW HARBINGER PUBLICATIONS

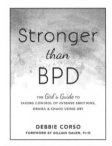

STRONGER THAN BPD

The Girl's Guide to Taking
Control of Intense Emotions,
Drama & Chaos Using DBT

978-1626254954 / US $16.95

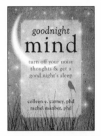

GOODNIGHT MIND

Turn Off Your Noisy Thoughts
& Get a Good Night's Sleep

978-1608826186 / US $17.95

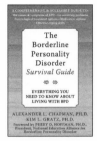

**THE BORDERLINE
PERSONALITY
SURVIVAL GUIDE**

Everything You Need to Know
About Living with BPD

978-1572245075 / US $17.95

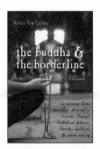

**THE BUDDHA &
THE BORDERLINE**

My Recovery from Borderline
Personality Disorder through
Dialectical Behavior Therapy,
Buddhism & Online Dating

978-1572247109 / US $18.95

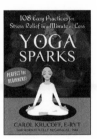

YOGA SPARKS

108 Easy Practices for Stress
Relief in a Minute or Less

978-1608827008 / US $16.95

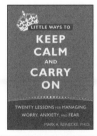

**LITTLE WAYS TO KEEP
CALM & CARRY ON**

Twenty Lessons for Managing
Worry, Anxiety & Fear

978-1572248816 / US $15.95

newharbingerpublications
1-800-748-6273 / newharbinger.com

(VISA, MC, AMEX / prices subject to change without notice)

Follow Us

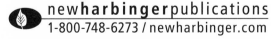

Don't miss out on new books in the subjects that interest you.
Sign up for our Book Alerts at **newharbinger.com/bookalerts**

FROM OUR PUBLISHER—

As the publisher at New Harbinger and a clinical psychologist since 1978, I know that emotional problems are best helped with evidence-based therapies. These are the treatments derived from scientific research (randomized controlled trials) that show what works. Whether these treatments are delivered by trained clinicians or found in a self-help book, they are designed to provide you with proven strategies to overcome your problem.

Therapies that aren't evidence-based—whether offered by clinicians or in books—are much less likely to help. In fact, therapies that aren't guided by science may not help you at all. That's why this New Harbinger book is based on scientific evidence that the treatment can relieve emotional pain.

This is important: if this book isn't enough, and you need the help of a skilled therapist, use the following resources to find a clinician trained in the evidence-based protocols appropriate for your problem. And if you need more support— a community that understands what you're going through and can show you ways to cope—resources for that are provided below, as well.

Real help is available for the problems you have been struggling with. The skills you can learn from evidence-based therapies will change your life.

Matthew McKay, PhD
Publisher, New Harbinger Publications

If you need a therapist, the following organization can help you find a therapist trained in dialectical behavior therapy (DBT).

Behavioral Tech, LLC
please visit www.behavioraltech.org and click on *Find a DBT Therapist.*

For additional support for patients, family, and friends, please contact the following:

National Alliance on Mental Illness (NAMI)
Please visit www.nami.org

BPD Central **Visit www.bpdcentral.org**

Treatment and Research Advancements Association for Personality Disorder (TARA)
Visit www.tara4bpd.org

Register your **new harbinger** titles for additional benefits!

When you register your **new harbinger** title—purchased in any format, from any source—you get access to benefits like the following:

- Downloadable accessories like printable worksheets and extra content

- Instructional videos and audio files

- Information about updates, corrections, and new editions

Not every title has accessories, but we're adding new material all the time.

Access free accessories in 3 easy steps:

1. Sign in at NewHarbinger.com (or **register** to create an account).

2. Click on **register a book**. Search for your title and click the **register** button when it appears.

3. Click on the **book cover or title** to go to its details page. Click on **accessories** to view and access files.

That's all there is to it!

If you need help, visit:

NewHarbinger.com/accessories

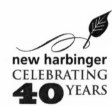

new harbinger
CELEBRATING
40 YEARS